Make You Healthy Again

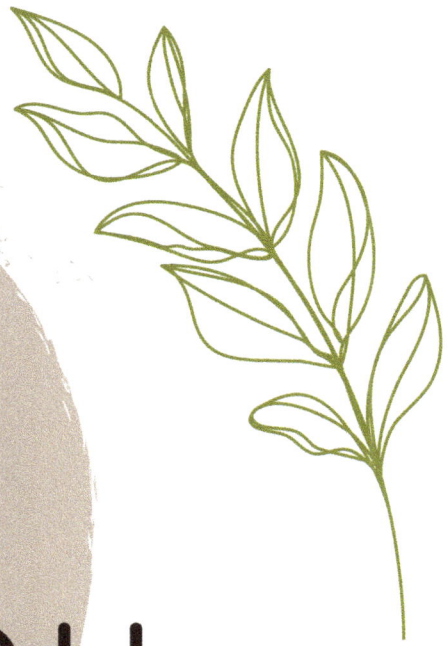

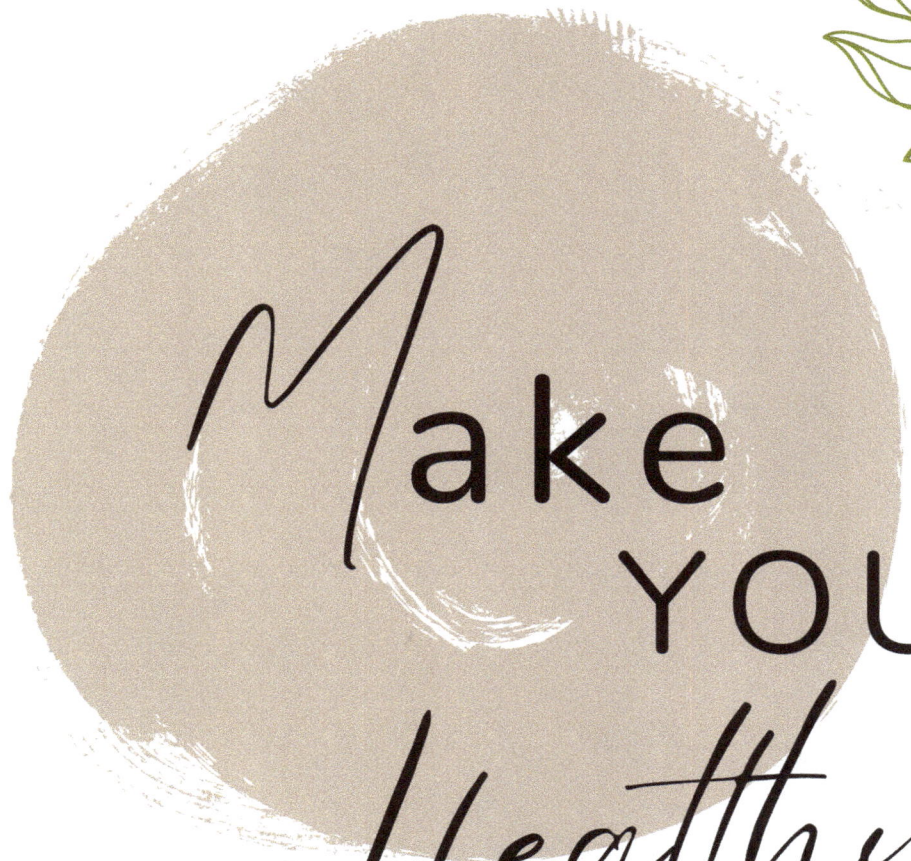

Make YOU Healthy Again

A PERSONAL ROAD MAP TO HEALING

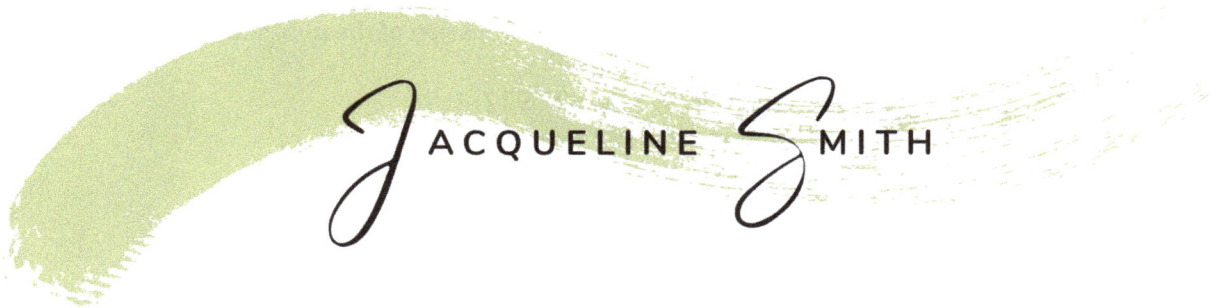

Jacqueline Smith

Make You Healthy Again
Jacqueline Smith
Copyright © 2024 by Supportive Gut Wellness Coaching LLC

ISBN: 979-8-218-55972-4
Published by: Supportive Gut Wellness Coaching LLC
New Smyrna Beach, FL

Printed in the United States of America

CONTENTS

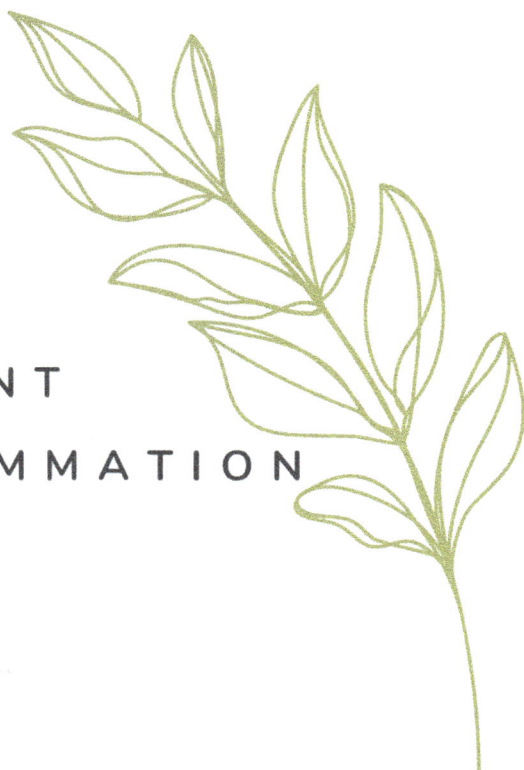

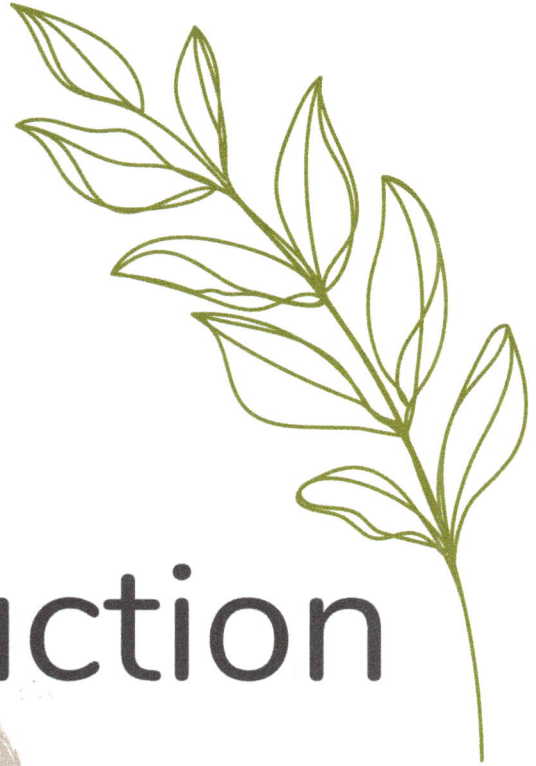

Introduction

Welcome

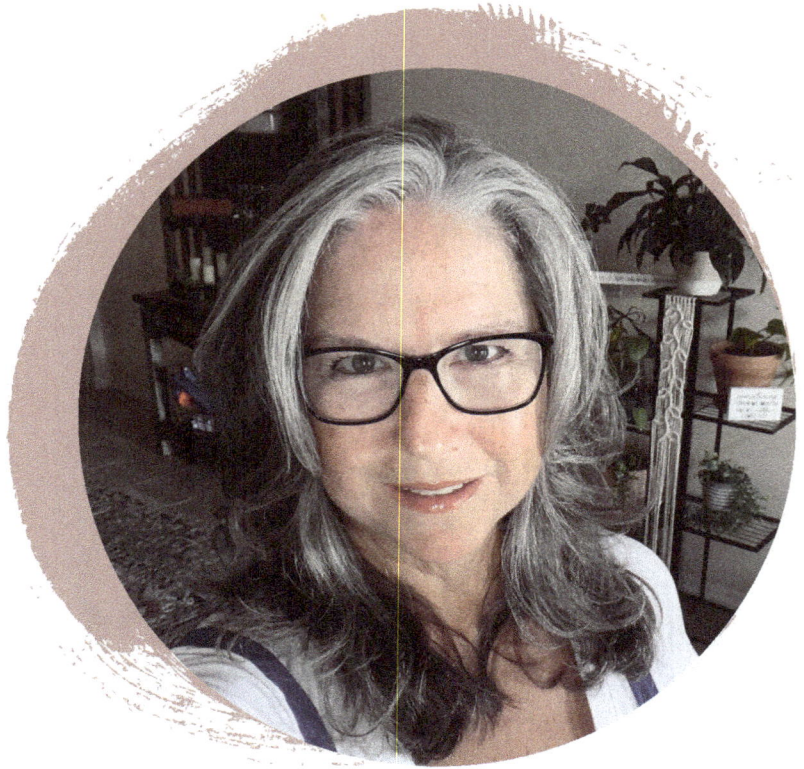

Hello!

I'm a certified functional nutrition coach passionate about guiding individuals on their journey to reclaim their health and well-being. By providing knowledge and guidance, I hope to help you make changes towards a healthy life.

This book is a guided workbook with questions and activities to help uncover the root causes of your illness and track your progress.

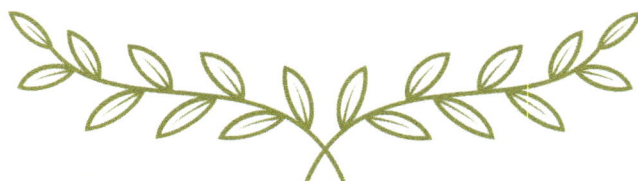

Introduction

My Story

After suffering from undiagnosed illnesses and watching family members endure the same, I became frustrated and tired of hearing, 'your blood work is normal,' or 'there's nothing wrong with you,' even though I felt sick all the time. Turning to functional nutrition, I experienced healing firsthand. As I introduced these tips and insights to others, I witnessed them embark on their journeys toward a healthier life.

Jacqueline R Smith

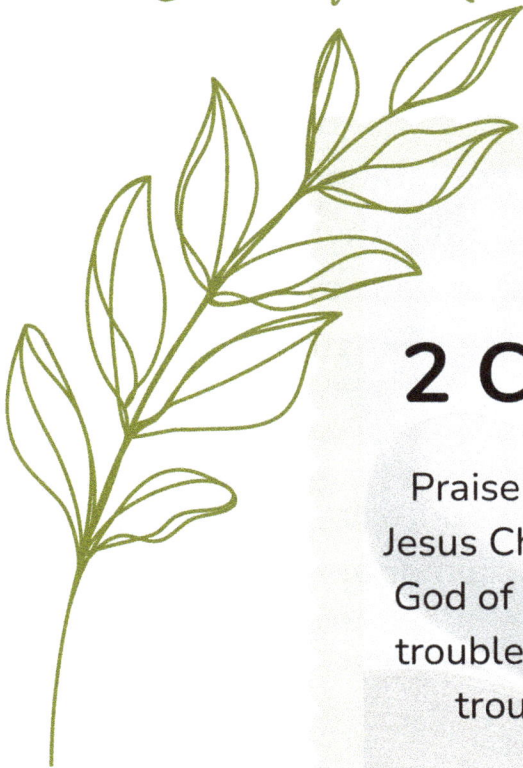

2 Corinthians 1:3-4

Praise be to the God and Father of our Lord Jesus Christ, the Father of compassion and the God of all comfort, who comforts us in all our troubles, so that we can comfort those in any trouble with the comfort we ourselves received from God.

God's Word

Discovery

This book is designed to guide you in discovering what your body needs for healing. Each section presents thought provoking questions, discovery activities, knowledgeable resources, and prompts to track your progress.

This is not intended to be read quickly, but rather worked through at your own pace, taking the next step when you are ready.

Before you begin, please read the disclaimer at the end.

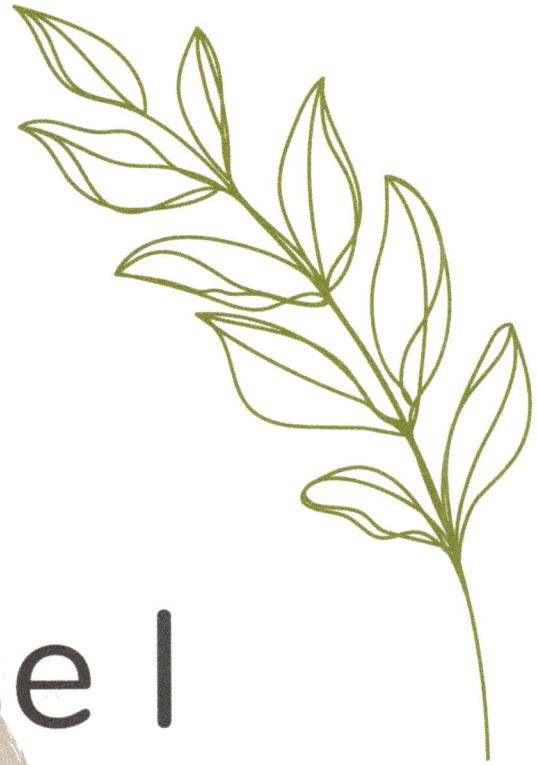

Phase I

Starting Point

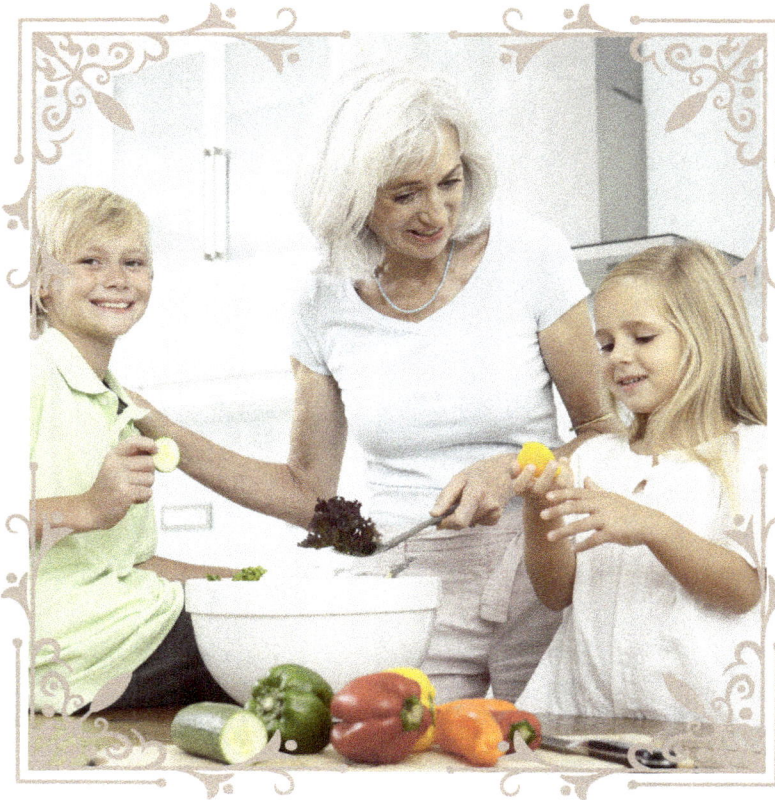

Find your Motivation

What is your goal? Why do you want to achieve it? Do you want to feel better? Do you want to spend more time with family? Are you trying to keep up with your grandkids?

Write down your goals and reasons, and refer to this page often throughout your journey.

YOUR GOAL:

_____

_____

_____

_____

_____

_____

_____

Your Motivation

About the Process

Do you wonder why certain 'cures' work for others but not for you? It's because we are all unique. What works for one person may not work for another. Together, we will find what works best for you.

Write down some things you've tried before that didn't work.

Revisit what you have tried in the past that worked.

DIDN'T WORK:

WORKED:

Symptom Check

When we begin to heal, it's easy to forget how we felt before we started. Let's track our symptoms. Check off the symptoms that best describe what you are currently experiencing regularly.

☐ Chronic Fatigue

☐ Unexplained Pain

☐ Digestive Issues

☐ Brain Fog

☐ Headaches and Migraines

☐ Skin Problems

☐ Sleep Disturbance

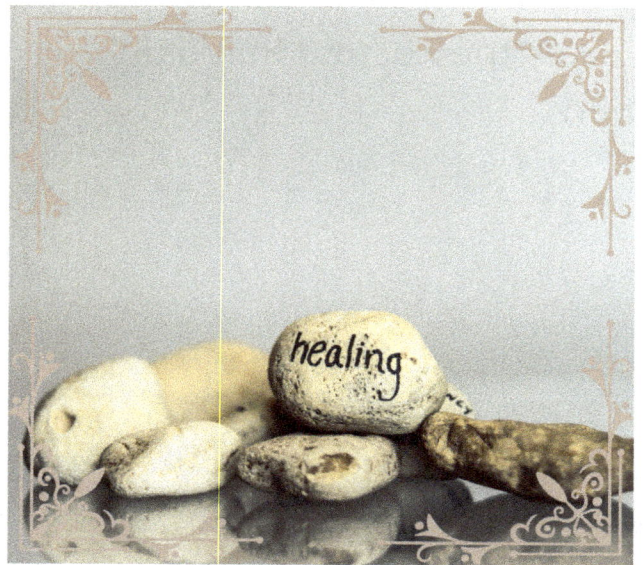

You are probably experiencing many more symptoms. Write those below

_____

_____

_____

Reflection Time

Be prayerful about your goals.

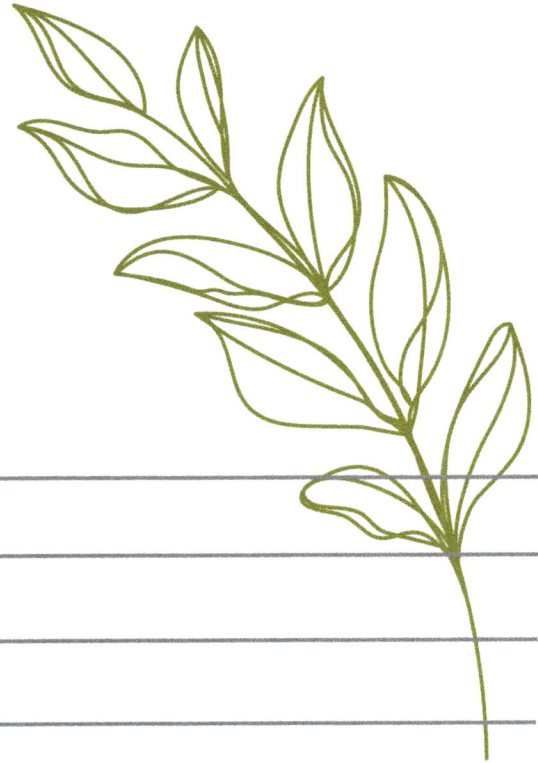

_____

_____

_____

_____

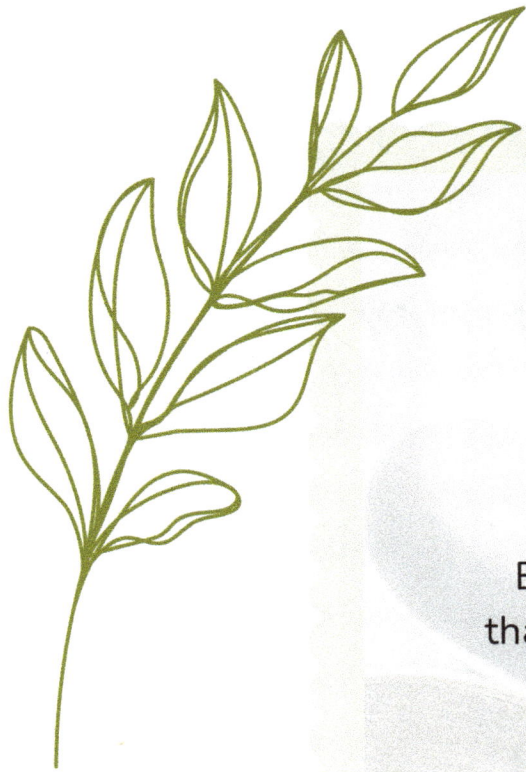

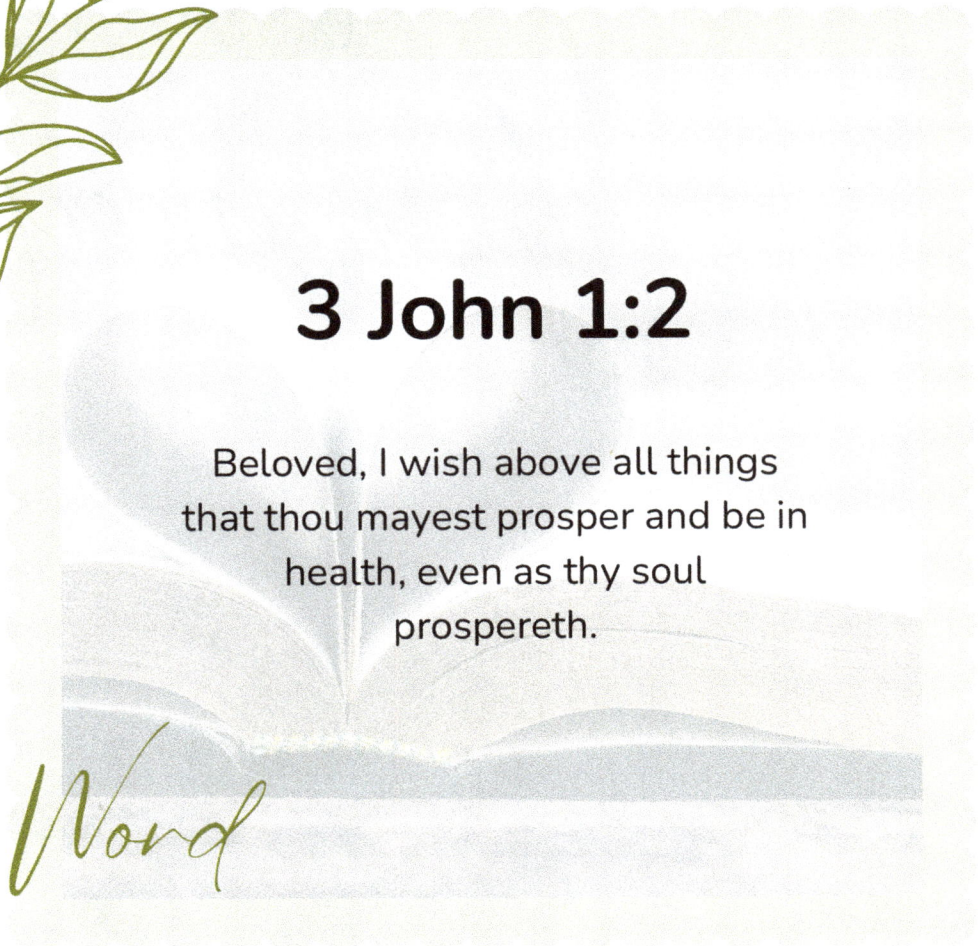

3 John 1:2

Beloved, I wish above all things that thou mayest prosper and be in health, even as thy soul prospereth.

God's Word

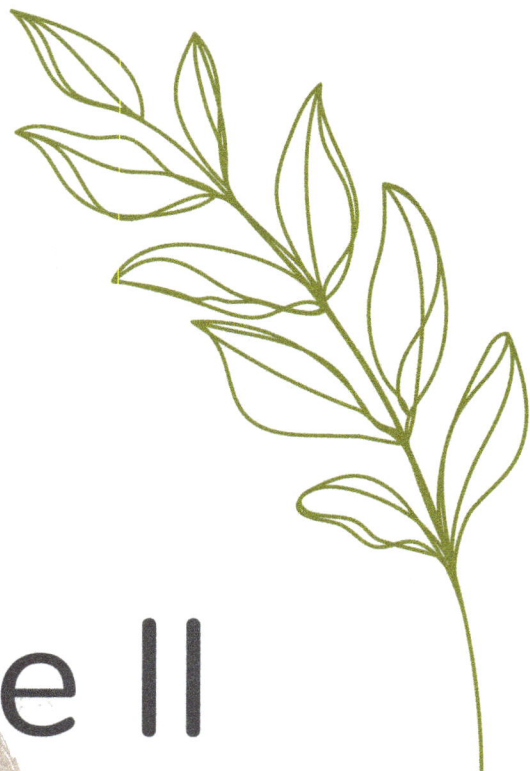

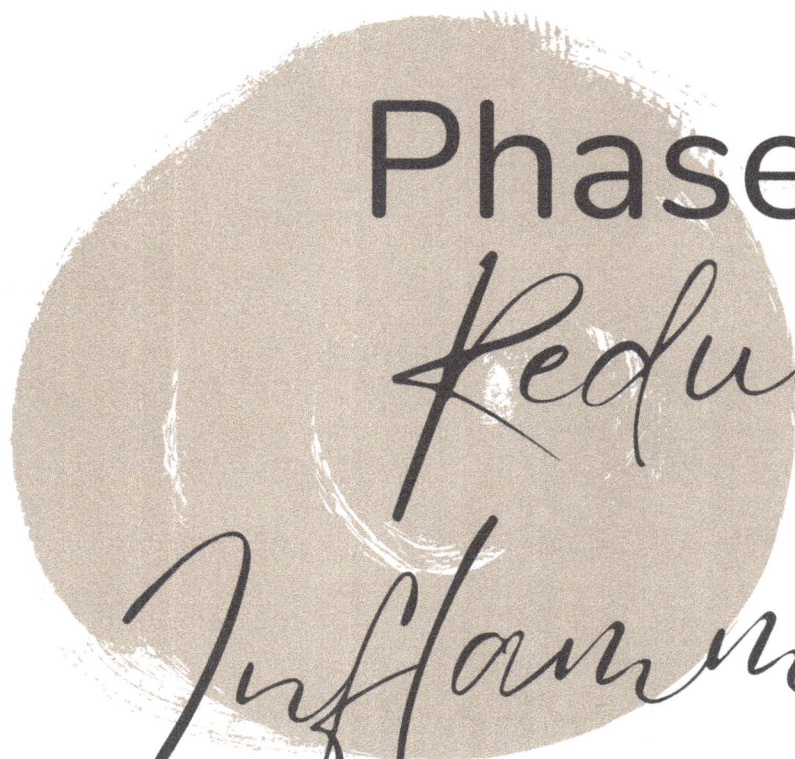

Phase II
Reduce Inflammation

If you checked any of the symptoms listed, you probably have inflammation.

Let's start by calming the inflammation.

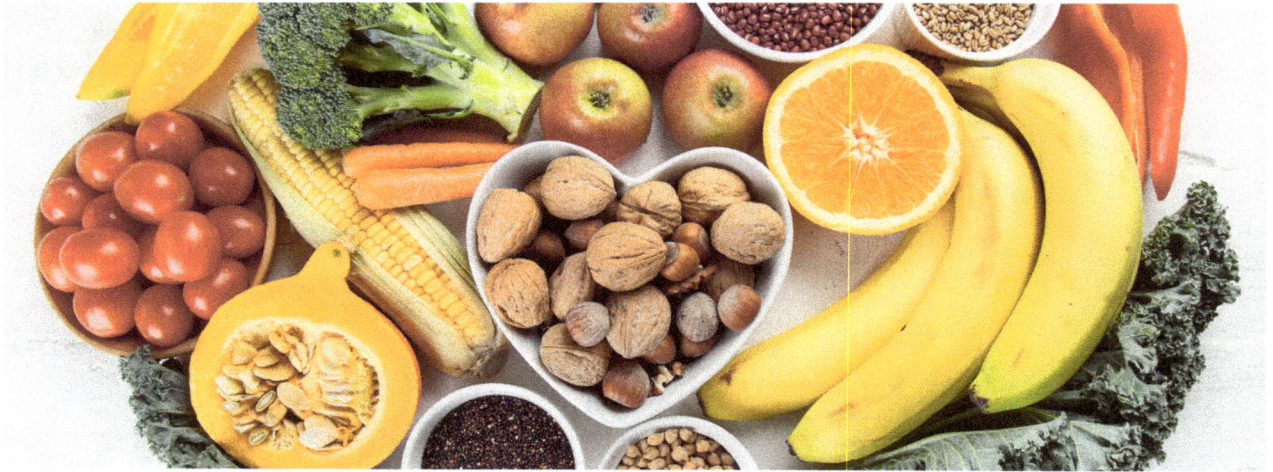

Long Term Goal Action Steps

1

Remove common inflammatory foods temporarily. These include processed foods, refined sugar, and gluten. Track how you feel.

2

After several days, review your tracking and document how you are feeling. Refer back to your symptom check page as a reminder.

3

Add gluten back into your diet but in the form of whole grains, not refined flour. Monitor your symptoms! If you feel worse, then remove it again.

"You want me to do what?"

Keep Reading

More Details...

When I shared these action steps with a dear friend, she said, 'You want me to give up sugar, gluten, and all that good stuff?' Giving up sugar, gluten, and processed foods all at once can be overwhelming, so we'll take it step by step. First, we'll learn what these foods are and why it's beneficial to remove them. Then, we'll begin removing a few things at a time, tracking how you feel along the way. Even after ten years of making small changes myself, I still have a few pantry items with added sugar. Progress takes time, and that's okay!

PROCESSED FOODS

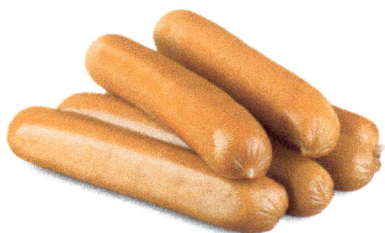

Processed foods are items that have been altered from their original state before reaching the consumer. These alterations often include the addition of preservatives, artificial flavors, colors, sweeteners, and other chemicals.

Additionally, some processed foods may contain ingredients derived from genetically modified organisms (GMOs).

GMOs are organisms whose genetic material has been altered in a way that does not occur naturally. In the context of food, this often involves the genetic modification of plants to enhance desired traits such as resistance to pests, diseases, or tolerance to herbicides.

Processed foods can include ready-to-eat meals, snacks, and beverages. While convenient, these foods may lack essential nutrients found in whole, unprocessed alternatives.

Heavily processed foods have been associated with health concerns, including nutritional imbalances and increased risk of certain chronic conditions.

Processed foods contain preservatives and additives made from chemical compounds.

Processed foods scale

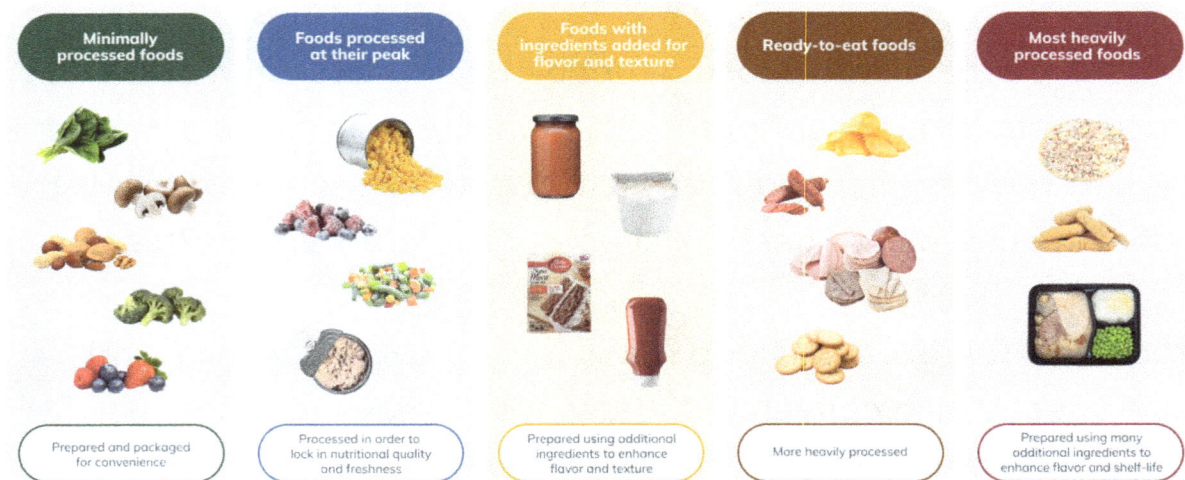

Minimally processed foods	Foods processed at their peak	Foods with ingredients added for flavor and texture	Ready-to-eat foods	Most heavily processed foods
Prepared and packaged for convenience	Processed in order to lock in nutritional quality and freshness	Prepared using additional ingredients to enhance flavor and texture	More heavily processed	Prepared using many additional ingredients to enhance flavor and shelf-life

W H Y ?

Preservatives and additives commonly found in processed foods include:

Artificial Sweeteners:

Substances like aspartame, saccharin, and sucralose are used to enhance sweetness without adding calories.

Artificial Colors:

Chemical compounds that provide color to food and drinks, such as Red 40, Yellow 5, and Blue 1.

Artificial Flavors:

Synthetic compounds used to mimic natural flavors, providing a specific taste to processed foods.

Emulsifiers:

Substances like lecithin and polysorbates help maintain the texture and consistency of processed foods.

Stabilizers:

Ingredients such as carrageenan and xanthan gum are used to prevent separation and maintain uniformity in certain products.

Preservatives:

Chemicals like sodium benzoate, BHA, and BHT are added to extend the shelf life of processed foods by inhibiting the growth of bacteria, yeast, and molds.

MSG (Monosodium Glutamate):

A flavor enhancer commonly used to add umami taste to processed foods.

High-Fructose Corn Syrup (HFCS):

A sweetener derived from corn used to sweeten many processed foods and beverages.

Agricultural chemicals, such as pesticides and herbicides, are used to protect crops from pests and diseases, ensuring a higher yield and preventing spoilage.

WHAT'S IN YOUR FOOD?

Let's look at just a couple of these to see what is hiding in our processed foods.

Ethyl methylphenylglycidate, also known as ethyl methyl phenyl glycidate or simply as "strawberry aldehyde," is a chemical compound commonly used in the production of artificial strawberry flavoring.

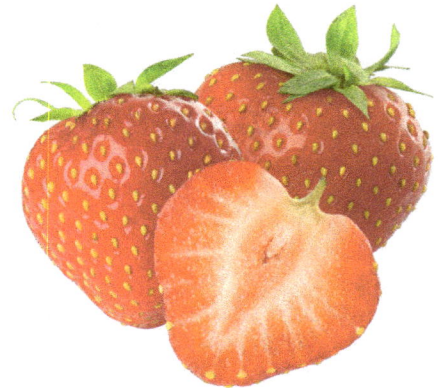

Ethyl methylphenylglycidate is responsible for imparting the characteristic sweet, fruity aroma and taste associated with ripe strawberries. It is synthesized in laboratories by chemically modifying other compounds to create a flavor that closely resembles natural strawberry flavor.

It is a synthetic compound, meaning it is not extracted from natural sources, but instead produced through chemical synthesis in laboratories. While the specific process for synthesizing ethyl methylphenylglycidate may vary, it typically involves starting with simpler chemical compounds and subjecting them to various chemical reactions to create the desired product.

One example of a product that may contain ethyl methylphenylglycidate is artificial strawberry flavoring, which is used in a wide range of food and beverage items such as candies, flavored beverages, yogurts, and desserts. While ethyl methylphenylglycidate may not always be explicitly listed on ingredient labels, it is often included as part of the "**natural flavors**" or "**artificial flavors**" category.

WHERE DO YOU THINK IT COMES FROM?

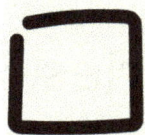 Crude Oil

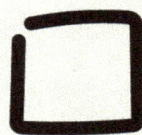 Strawberries

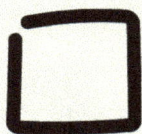 Coconut Oil

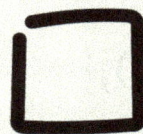 Beeswax

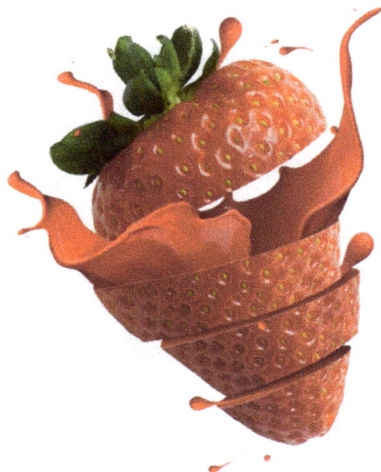

ANSWER

Many of the basic building blocks for synthetic organic chemicals, like phenylacetaldehyde (a key precursor for ethyl methylphenylglycidate), are derived from benzene, ethylene, or toluene, which are petrochemical products. These are obtained from the refining of crude oil or natural gas.

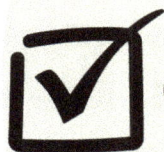 Crude Oil

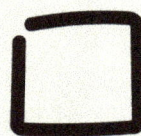 Strawberries

 Coconut Oil

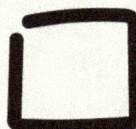 Beeswax

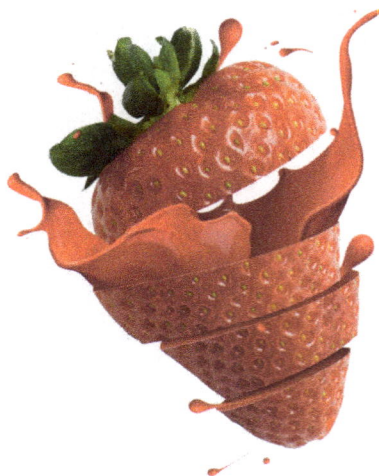

FD&C RED NO. 40 (ALLURA RED AC)

Allura Red is also typically synthesized from petroleum-derived compounds. It is used extensively in the food and beverage industry to color a wide range of products, including candies, soft drinks, desserts, snacks, sauces, and processed foods.

While Allura Red is approved for use as a food additive by regulatory agencies such as the U.S. Food and Drug Administration (FDA) and the European Food Safety Authority (EFSA), its safety has been the subject of some controversy. Some studies have suggested potential health concerns associated with Allura Red consumption, including allergic reactions and hyperactivity in children.

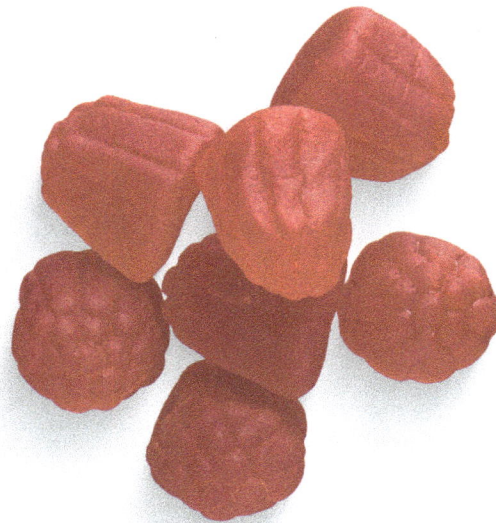

BHA AND BHT

BHA and BHT are preservatives, and both are also typically synthesized from petroleum-derived compounds. These chemicals are found in:

Processed Meats

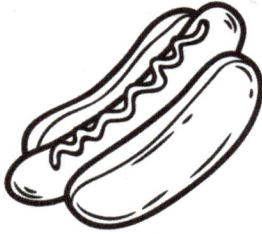

Breakfast Cereal

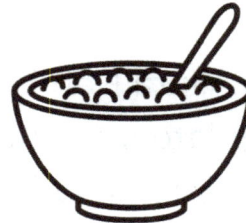

Chewing Gum

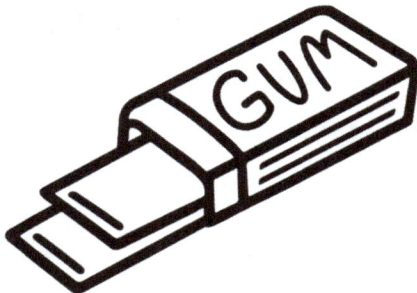

Nutritional Supplements

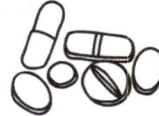

Cosmetics and Personal Care Products

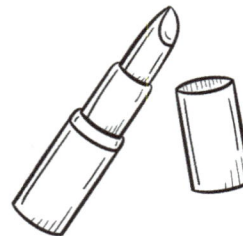

Baked Goods

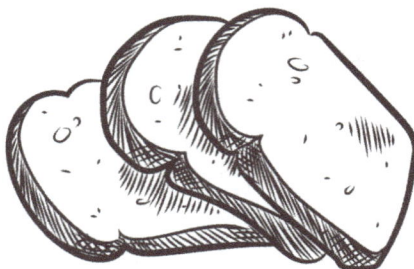

Snacks

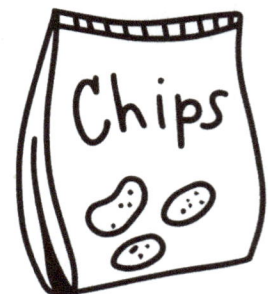

SUGAR

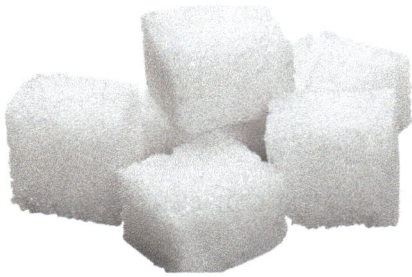

Added sugars are prevalent in many foods, and are used to enhance shelf life, increase palatability, increase energy, and satisfy consumer preference.

" Every time you eat or drink, you are either feeding disease or fighting it.
- Heather Morgan "

ARE YOU FEEDING DISEASE OR FIGHTING DISEASE?

These chemicals and sugars are linked to several health concerns including endocrine disruption and organ system toxicity.

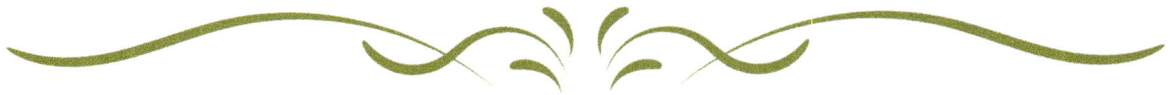

The chemicals, sugars, unhealthy fats, and artificial ingredients in processed foods cause the following health issues. Check which ones you are currently fighting:

- ☐ Obesity
- ☐ Type 2 Diabetes
- ☐ Heart Disease
- ☐ Cancer
- ☐ Digestive Issues

- ☐ Food Allergies /Sensitivities
- ☐ Neurological Disorders
- ☐ Metabolic Syndrome
- ☐ Dental Issues
- ☐ Non-Alcoholic Fatty Liver Disease

Symptom Check

Let's revisit symptoms. These are symptoms that you may experience from eating processed foods. Which ones are you experiencing?

☐ Heachaches

☐ Fatigue

☐ Bloating, Gas, Diarrhea

☐ Joint Pain

☐ Mood Swings, Irritability

☐ Skin Problems

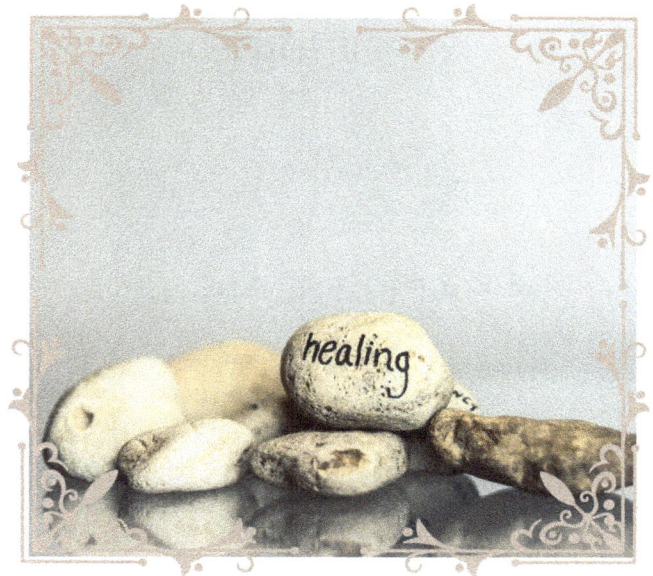

☐ Brain Fog, Memory Issues

☐ Inflammation

☐ Constipation, Abdominal discomfort

☐ Respiratory Symptoms (wheezing, coughing)

Multiple Choice

QUIZ

WHICH FOODS LISTED BELOW ARE PROCESSED?

A. APPLES

B. APPLE JUICE

C. APPLE SAUCE

D. CONVENIENT APPLE SLICE PACKAGES

WHAT IS THE MAIN PURPOSE OF PROCESSING FOODS?

A. TO REDUCE SPOILAGE AND EXTEND SHELF LIFE

B. TO INCREASE NUTRITIONAL CONTENT

C. TO REDUCE COST

WHICH OF THE FOLLOWING IS NOT A POTENTIAL HEALTH CONCERN ASSOCIATED WITH CONSUMING PROCESSED FOODS?

A. OBESITY

B. TYPE 2 DIABETES

C. IMPROVE DIGESTION

D. HEART DISEASE

ANSWERS

WHICH FOODS LISTED BELOW ARE PROCESSED?

A. APPLES

B. APPLE JUICE

C. APPLE SAUCE

D. CONVENIENT APPLE SLICE PACKAGES

WHAT IS THE MAIN PURPOSE OF PROCESSING FOODS?

A. TO REDUCE SPOILAGE AND EXTEND SHELF LIFE

B. TO INCREASE NUTRITIONAL CONTENT

C. TO REDUCE COST

WHICH OF THE FOLLOWING IS NOT A POTENTIAL HEALTH CONCERN ASSOCIATED WITH CONSUMING PROCESSED FOODS?

A. OBESITY

B. TYPE 2 DIABETES

C. IMPROVE DIGESTION

D. HEART DISEASE

FEEDBACK

WHICH FOODS LISTED BELOW ARE PROCESSED?

A. APPLES

B. APPLE JUICE

C. APPLE SAUCE

D. CONVENIENT APPLE
    SLICE PACKAGES

Apple juices, applesauce, and even those convenient apple slice packages are all considered processed.

NOTE: Just because these are processed, does not necessarily mean they are bad.
What are the added ingredients, if any?
Are there added sugars?
Are there added chemicals to preserve them longer, enhance the taste or improve the color?

WHAT IS THE MAIN PURPOSE OF PROCESSING FOODS?

A. TO REDUCE SPOILAGE AND EXTEND SHELF LIFE

B. TO INCREASE NUTRITIONAL CONTENT

C. TO REDUCE COST

The main purpose of processing foods is to reduce spoilage and extend shelf life.

Other purposes for processed foods are convenience, increasing accessibility, enhancing flavors or textures. The problems associated with processed foods are both the processing, which degrades food quality, and what is being added.

WHICH OF THE FOLLOWING IS **NOT** A POTENTIAL HEALTH CONCERN ASSOCIATED WITH CONSUMING PROCESSED FOODS?

A. OBESITY

B. TYPE 2 DIABETES

C. IMPROVE DIGESTION

D. HEART DISEASE

Obesity, Type 2 Diabetes and Heart Disease are all potential health concerns associated with consuming processed foods.

GLUTEN

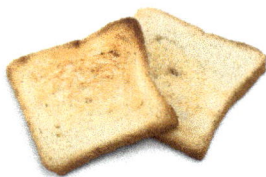

Gluten is a protein found in grain. Not everyone needs to be gluten-free, but you can support your digestive system by choosing whole grains over white flour.

Maybe you have cut out breads to remove gluten from your diet, but still experience symptoms. Identifying gluten-containing foods can be crucial for those following a gluten-free diet. Gluten is commonly found in:

Wheat Products: This includes items like bread, pasta, couscous, and baked goods.

Barley and Rye: Certain products made from barley and rye, such as malt, beer, and some types of cereal, can contain gluten.

Oats (if Contaminated): While oats themselves are gluten-free, they may be contaminated during processing. Look for certified gluten-free oats.

Processed Foods: Many processed foods may contain hidden gluten, such as sauces, soups, and processed meats.

Thickening Agents: Some sauces and gravies use wheat flour as a thickening agent.

Snack Foods: Items like pretzels, crackers, and certain snack bars may contain gluten.

Dressings and Sauces: Salad dressings, soy sauce, and marinades might have gluten-containing ingredients.

Always read food labels carefully, and when in doubt, choose products labeled as "gluten-free." Additionally, fresh fruits, vegetables, most dairy products, and naturally gluten-free grains like rice and quinoa are safe options.

Why Remove Gluten:

Many wonder why we target gluten in dietary changes. Gluten, found in wheat, barley, and rye, can trigger various health issues. Let's dive into the details to understand the impact of gluten on our bodies and explore healthier alternatives for a balanced and thriving lifestyle.

To deepen your understanding, let's explore a visual guide. The chart below, courtesy of the Functional Nutrition Lab, illustrates various disorders associated with gluten. This comprehensive view will shed light on the spectrum of gluten-related issues.

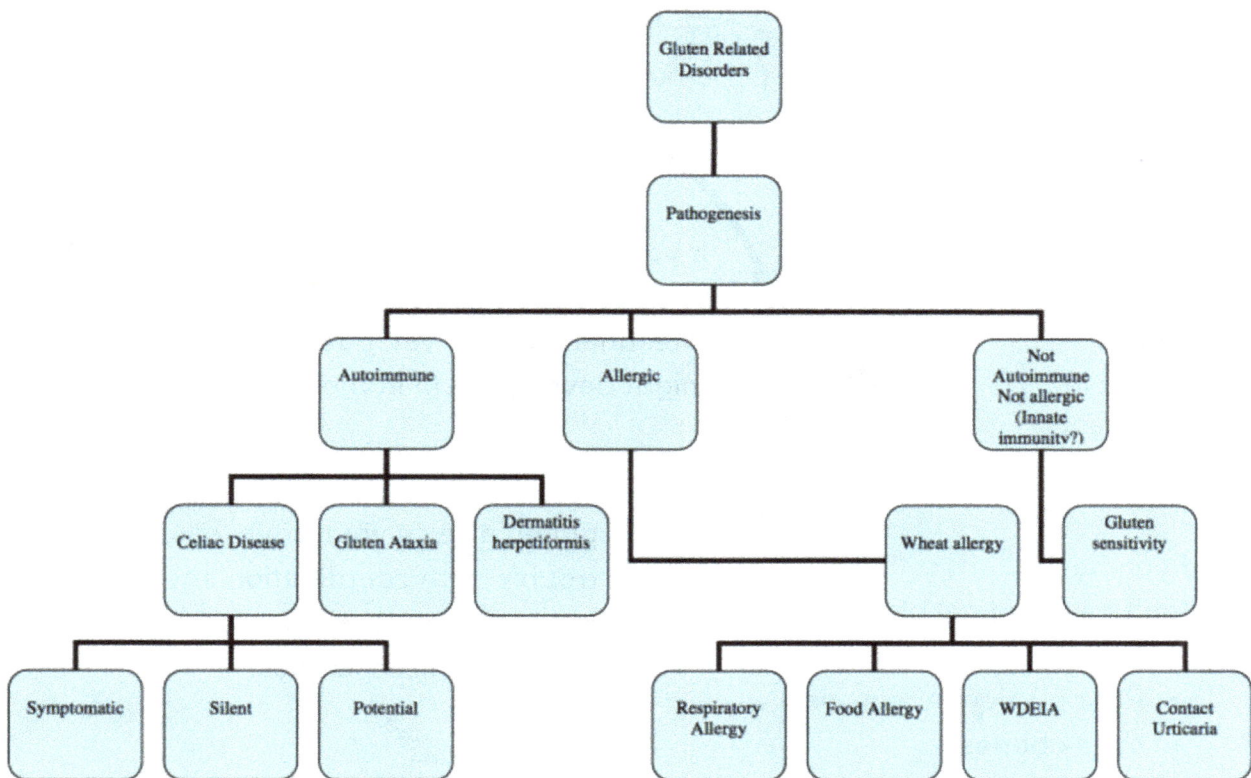

```
                    Gluten Related
                       Disorders
                           |
                      Pathogenesis
                           |
        _____|_____
       |                   |                   |
   Autoimmune          Allergic          Not Autoimmune
                                          Not allergic
                                            (Innate
                                           immunity?)
       |                                    |
  _____|_____                  _____|_____
 |        |         |                 |          |
Celiac  Gluten   Dermatitis       Wheat allergy  Gluten
Disease Ataxia  herpetiformis                   sensitivity
 |                                    |
_|_____                  _____|_____
|    |     |                |       |       |        |
Symptomatic Silent Potential Respiratory Food  WDEIA Contact
                            Allergy    Allergy      Urticaria
```

Pathogensis

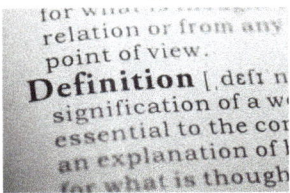

What is Pathogenesis? Pathogenesis is how a disease starts and gets worse in the body. It includes all the steps of how a disease begins, grows, and affects the body. If it's an autoimmune disease, it might be related to gluten.

Let's break down the conditions linked to gluten:

Celiac disease occurs when the small intestines have been damaged from eating gluten. This makes it hard for your body to absorb nutrients from food.

If you have symptomatic celiac disease, you have noticeable symptoms like:

- Diarrhea
- Stomach pain
- Bloating
- Constipation
- Fatigue
- Weight loss
- Anemia
- Skin rash
- Joint pain
- Neurological issues

If you have silent celiac disease, you don't have noticeable symptoms, but can still have problems like:
- Poor nutrient absorption
- Weak bones
- Fertility issues
- Nerve problems
- Higher risk of certain cancers

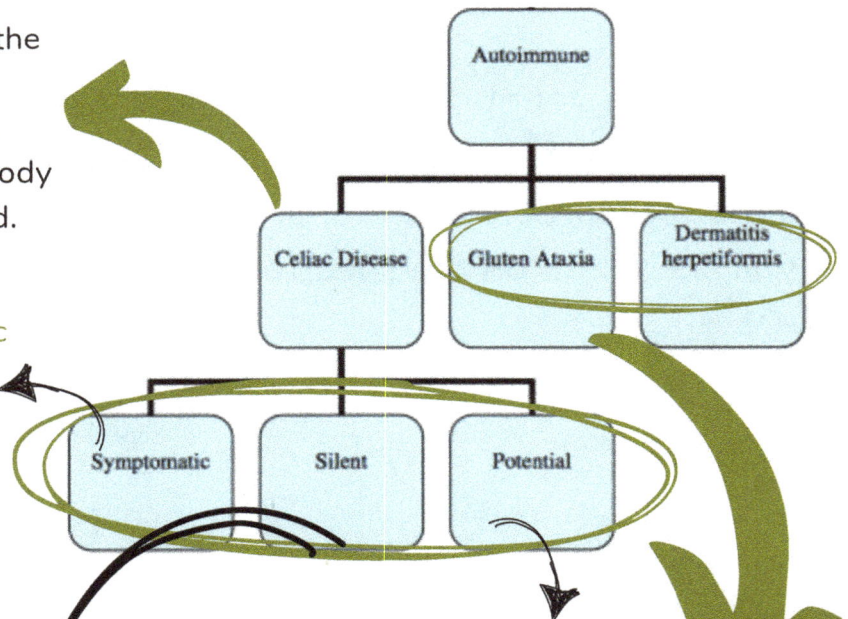

If you have potential celiac disease, you don't have symptoms or intestinal damage yet, but you might develop them in the future.

Gluten ataxia is a condition where gluten affects your brain, causing trouble with coordination and balance, but it doesn't damage your intestines like celiac disease does.

Dermatitis herpetiformis is a skin condition with itchy, blistering rashes caused by eating gluten. It's often linked to celiac disease.

Allergy:

If it is determined that you do not have celiac disease, then it may be an allergy to wheat.

If someone is allergic to wheat, a respiratory allergy means they may experience symptoms such as nasal congestion, sneezing, coughing, wheezing, and shortness of breath when exposed to wheat particles or wheat dust, especially in occupational settings like bakeries or flour mills.

If someone is allergic to wheat, a food allergy means they can experience symptoms such as hives, itching, swelling, digestive issues, and in severe cases, anaphylaxis, when they consume wheat or foods containing wheat.

Allergic

Wheat allergy

Respiratory Allergy   Food Allergy   WDEIA   Contact Urticaria

Stands for "Wheat-Dependent Exercise-Induced Anaphylaxis." This is a rare condition where an individual experiences anaphylaxis when consuming wheat and engaging in physical exercise afterward. It's a specific subtype of wheat allergy that requires careful management and avoidance of wheat consumption before physical activity.

Contact urticaria in the context of a wheat allergy means that direct contact with wheat or wheat-containing products can cause localized hives or skin rash at the contact site.

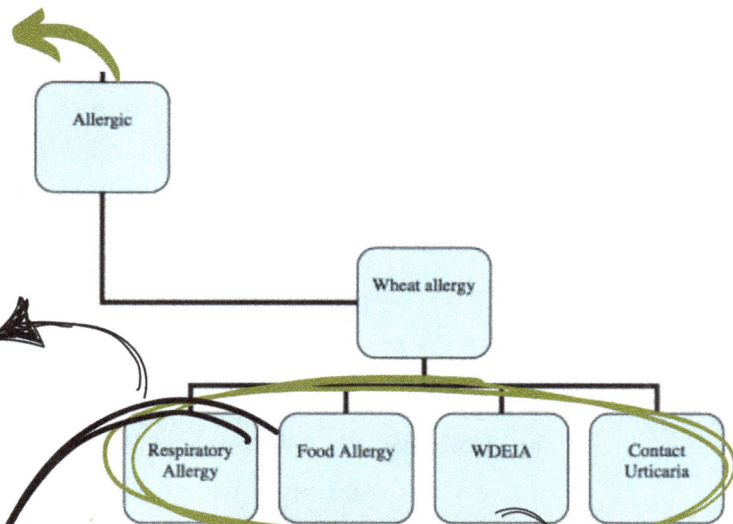

Non Autoimmune/Not Allergic:

If you do not have an autoimmune disease or allergy to wheat, you could still be gluten-sensitive.

People with a sensitivity to gluten may experience symptoms such as bloating, abdominal pain, diarrhea, constipation, fatigue, headaches, joint pain, and skin problems after consuming gluten-containing foods. These symptoms are similar to those of celiac disease but are typically less severe and do not involve the characteristic intestinal damage seen in celiac disease.

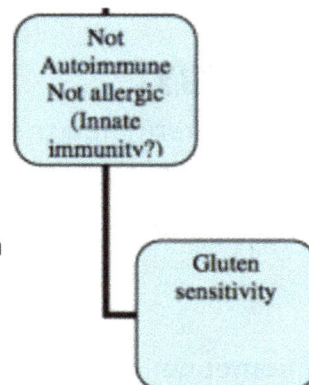

Not Autoimmune Not allergic (Innate immunity?)

Gluten sensitivity

This gluten intolerance can be frustrating because it is as if the tolerance level for gluten shifts. One day you might feel fine after eating that delicious bread and the next time, you are doubled over in pain.

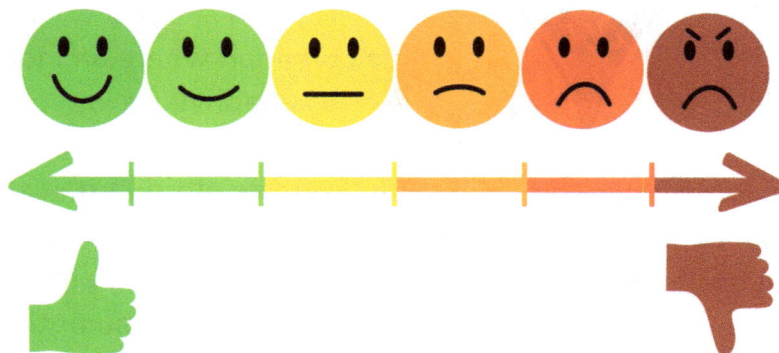

Factors such as stress, overall health, and the amount of gluten consumed can influence how someone reacts to gluten-containing foods. Therefore, while someone may tolerate small amounts of gluten on occasion, they may experience symptoms if they consume larger amounts or if their overall health changes.

what will you remove?

Pick a few items from each category to remove from your diet.

Processed:

Sugars:

Gluten:

REMOVE:

You Got This!

Track It!

Feel free to use the lines on this page to jot down your symptoms, mood, or anything else that comes to mind— or you could even doodle it!

still some pain

brain fog better

rash

Symptoms

less headaches

need sleep

swelling gone

Track It

Reflection Time

Removing the chemicals found in processed foods will help your body function better. What else do you need to remove from your life?

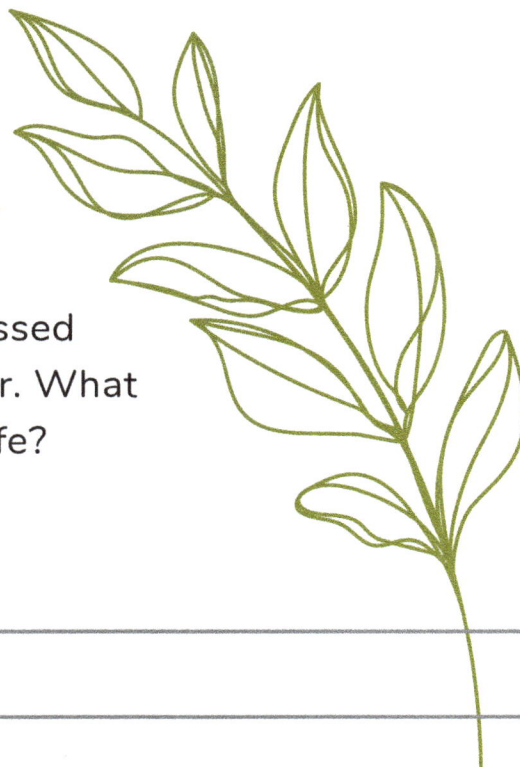

_____

_____

_____

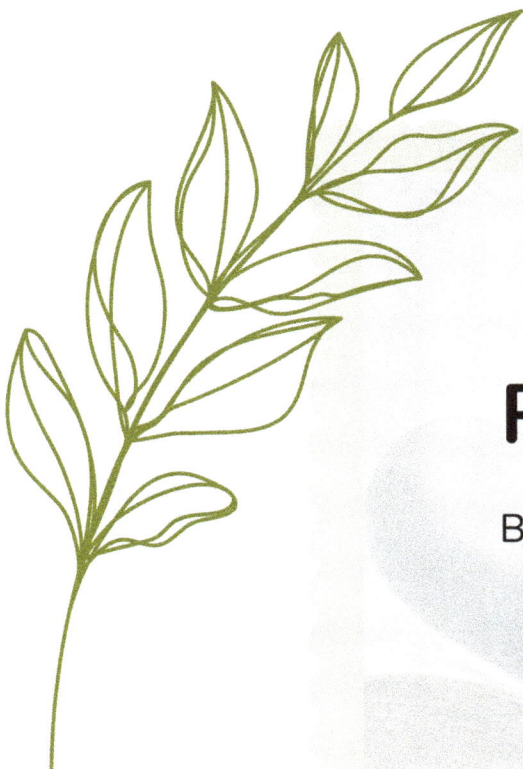

Proverbs 3:7-8

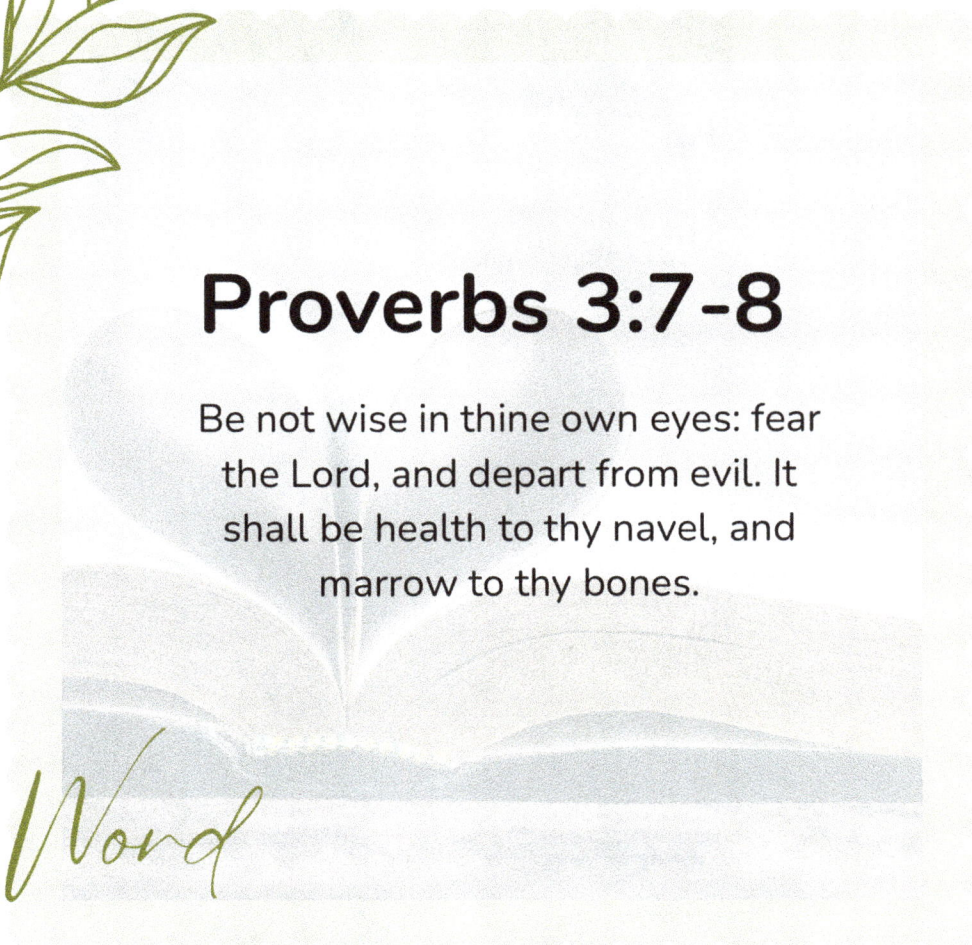

Be not wise in thine own eyes: fear the Lord, and depart from evil. It shall be health to thy navel, and marrow to thy bones.

God's Word

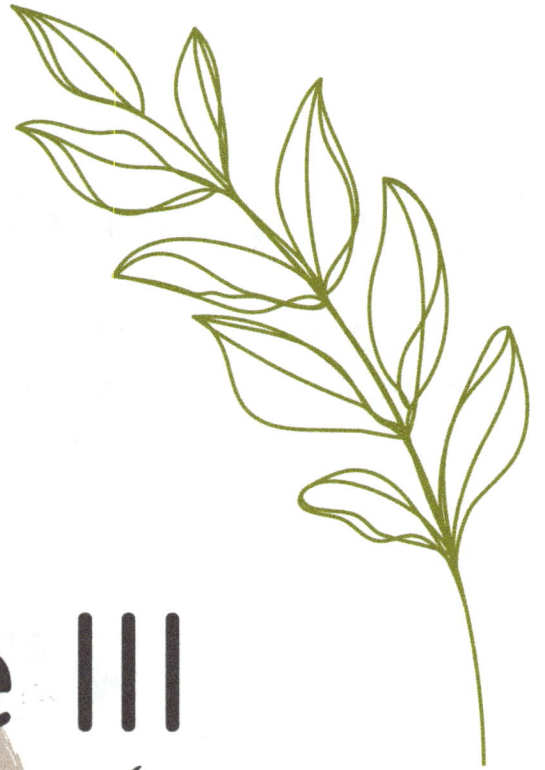

Phase III

New Ways

SHIFT YOUR
thought

FROM
"What do I eat"

TO
"Why do I eat"

Old Way vs. New Way

Rather than focusing on what we cannot have, let's think about replacing foods. We are going to take out the bad and replace it with good. Then let's look at why we eat these new foods.

THEN

NOW

Processed Foods:
frozen meals, prepackaged snacks, instant noodles, deli meats, canned foods with preservatives, soft drinks, chips

Whole Foods
Whole Grains
Pure Sweeteners:
fresh fruits, frozen fruit, dried fruits, fresh vegetables, quinoa, brown rice, millet, steal cut oats, buckwheat, nuts, seeds, legumes, nut butter, raw honey, 100% maple syrup,

VS.

Refined Sugar:
donuts, cookies, sodas, candy, processed snacks, condiments, ice cream, cereals

Gluten:
bread, pasta, crackers, cookies, sauces, gravy, beer, season blends

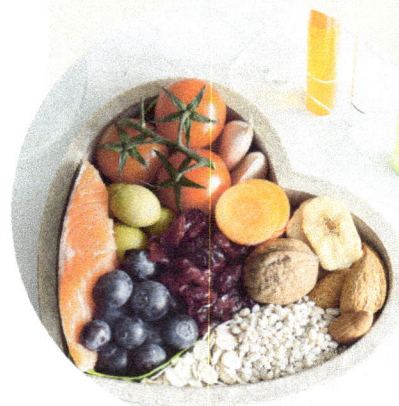

More Details...

Here is more information to guide you to foods that will support your healing journey.

ANTI INFLAMMATORY FOODS

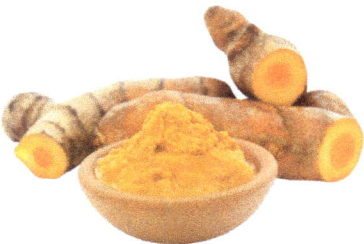

Most illnesses stem from inflammation. What foods can you ADD to your diet to help reduce inflammation?

Anti-inflammatory foods refer to foods that are believed to help reduce inflammation in the body. Inflammation is a natural response by the immune system to injury or infection, but chronic inflammation is associated with various health conditions such as heart disease, arthritis, and certain cancers.

Anti-inflammatory foods typically include fruits, vegetables, whole grains, nuts, seeds, fatty fish (like salmon and mackerel), and healthy fats (like olive oil and avocado). These foods are rich in antioxidants, vitamins, minerals, and phytonutrients that have been shown to have anti-inflammatory properties.

ANTI-INFLAMMATORY FOODS

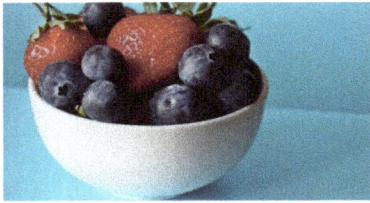

Berries

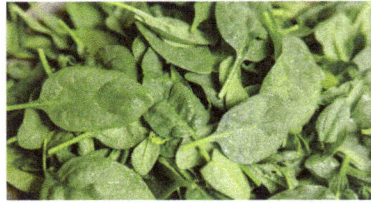

Leafy Greens

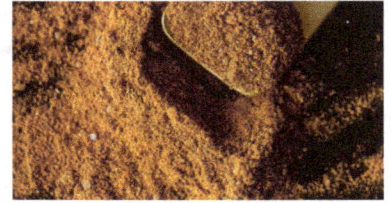

Turmeric

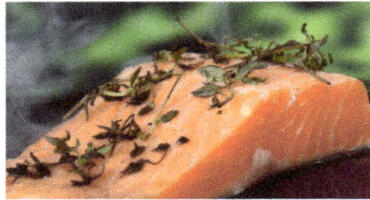

Fatty Fish

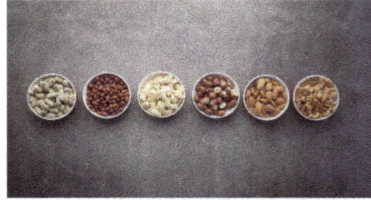

Nuts and Seeds

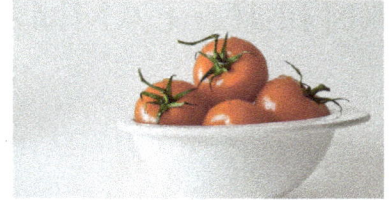

Tomatoes

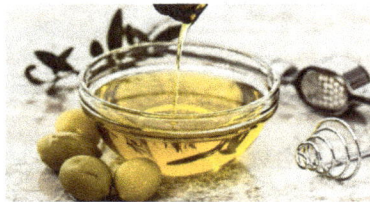

Olive Oil

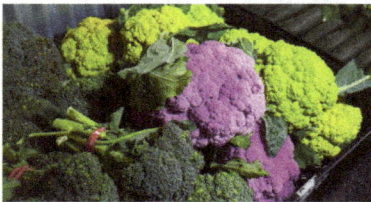

Cruciferous

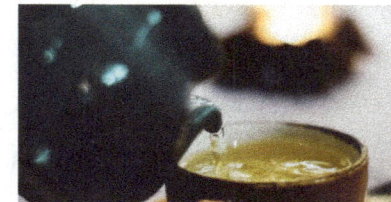

Green Tea

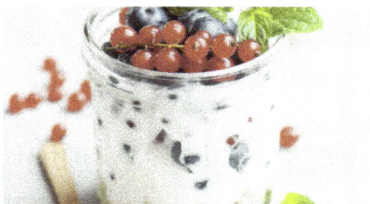

Probiotic Rich

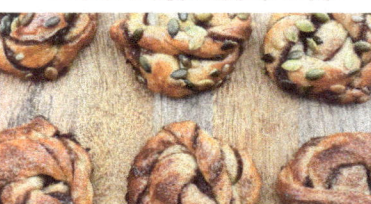

Whole Grains

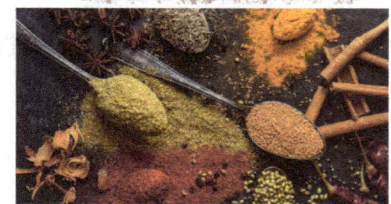

Spices

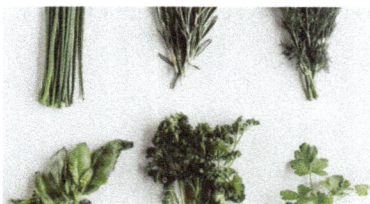

Herbs

Incorporating a variety of these anti-inflammatory foods into your diet can help promote overall health and reduce the risk of inflammation-related diseases. It's essential to maintain a balanced and diverse diet to ensure you're getting a wide range of nutrients and bioactive compounds.

WHOLE FOODS

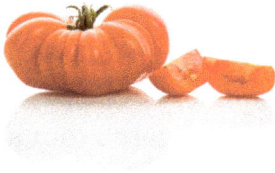

What was its life like before it presented itself to you for consumption? Foods that are in boxes can be mysterious. The life journey of whole foods are easier to imagine. To determine whether a food is whole or not, consider these questions.

Can I Imagine it Growing?

It is easy to picture a vegetable garden or apple on a tree. It's tough to picture a field of marshmallows. There are no streams where one can scoop out a bucket of soda, and no trees where you can pick Cheerios.

How Many Ingredients Does It Have?

A whole food has only one ingredient - itself. No label of ingredients is necessary on simple foods like avocados, salmon, and wild rice.

What's Been Done to the Food Since it's Been Harvested?

The less, the better. Many foods we eat no longer resemble anything found in nature. Stripped, refined, bleached, injected, hydrogenated, chemically treated, irradiated, and gassed, modern foods have had the life taken out of them. Read the list of ingredients on the label; if you can't pronounce something or can't imagine it growing, don't eat it. If it's not something that you could make in your kitchen or grow in your garden, be wary. For example, you can make miso (with some effort) from soybeans, but you can't make isolated soy protein.

Is the product "part" of a food or the "whole" entity?

Juice is only a part of a fruit.
Oil is only part of the olive.
Low-fat milk is only part of the milk.
When you eat a lot of partial foods, your body in its natural wisdom will crave the parts it didn't get.

How long has this food been known to nourish human beings?

Time and again, the rush to put a new drug, supplement, or food additive on the market has had questionable long-term effects. Most whole foods have been on the table for centuries.

Why?
Eating whole foods is beneficial for numerous reasons, contributing to overall health and well-being. Here are some of the key benefits:

Nutrient Density
Rich in Nutrients: Whole foods, such as fruits, vegetables, whole grains, nuts, seeds, and lean proteins, are packed with essential vitamins, minerals, and antioxidants that are vital for maintaining good health.

Balanced Nutrition: These foods provide a balanced mix of macronutrients (carbohydrates, proteins, fats) and micronutrients (vitamins and minerals), which help in various bodily functions.

Health Benefits
Disease Prevention: Diets rich in whole foods have been linked to a lower risk of chronic diseases such as heart disease, diabetes, and certain cancers. The fiber, antioxidants, and anti-inflammatory compounds in these foods help protect against illness.

Weight Management: Whole foods are often lower in calories and higher in fiber compared to processed foods, which can help maintain a healthy weight and prevent obesity.

Improved Digestion: The fiber content in whole foods promotes healthy digestion and regular bowel movements, reducing the risk of digestive issues like constipation and diverticulitis.

Better Energy Levels
Stable Energy: Whole foods, especially those rich in complex carbohydrates and proteins, provide a slow and steady release of energy, helping to maintain stable blood sugar levels and preventing energy crashes.

Enhanced Taste and Satisfaction
Natural Flavors: Whole foods are naturally flavorful and satisfying, often reducing the need for added sugars, salts, and unhealthy fats found in processed foods.

Mindful Eating: Eating whole foods encourages mindful eating practices, as these foods often require more preparation and consumption time, enhancing the overall eating experience.

Avoiding Harmful Additives
Reduced Additives: Whole foods are free from artificial additives, preservatives, and unhealthy trans fats commonly found in processed foods, which can have adverse health effects.

TIPS FOR INCORPORATING

Start with small changes

Focus on whole foods

Eat the rainbow

Plan your meals

Shop the perimeter of the grocery store

Add leafy greens

Use healthy fats

Spice it up

Snack smart

Stay hydrated

Read labels

Choose grass-fed meats

By incorporating these tips into your daily routine, you can gradually increase your intake of anti-inflammatory foods and enjoy the health benefits they offer. Remember to listen to your body and make choices that work best for you.

UNDERSTANDING FOOD LABELS

Chances are, you're already familiar with the basics of reading a nutritional label. But let's take a moment to refresh our understanding. Sometimes, we need a quick reminder to ensure we're making the best choices for our health.

Serving Size: This tells you the amount of food considered one serving, and all the information on the label is based on this serving size.

Calories: This indicates the number of calories in one serving of the food.

Macronutrients: Look for the amounts of these macronutrients:

- Fats: Total fat, saturated fat, trans fat, and cholesterol.
- Carbohydrates: Total carbohydrates, dietary fiber, sugars, and added sugars (if applicable).
- Proteins: The amount of protein per serving.
- Sodium: The quantity of sodium present in the food item.

1
2
3
4
5

Nutrition Facts Valeur nutritive		
Per 1 cup (250 mL) / par 1 tasse (250 mL)		
Amount Teneur		**% Daily Value** % valeur quotidienne
Calories / Calories 80		
Fat / Lipides 0 g		0 %
Saturated / saturés 0 g + Trans / trans 0 g		0 %
Cholesterol / Cholestérol 0 mg		
Sodium / Sodium 115 mg		5 %
Carbohydrate / Glucides 12 g		4 %
Fibre / Fibres 0 g		0 %
Sugars / Sucres 11 g		
Protein / Protéines 9 g		
Vitamin A / Vitamine A		15 %
Vitamin C / Vitamine C		0 %
Calcium / Calcium		30 %
Iron / Fer		0 %
Vitamin D / Vitamine D		45 %

Micronutrients: Check for the presence and amount of vitamins and minerals, typically listed as a percentage of the recommended daily value (DV).

Sugars: Make note of the amount of sugar. We will need to review the ingredients to determine where the sugar is coming from. We want to avoid "added sugars".

Macronutrients:

✔ COMPLEX CARBS

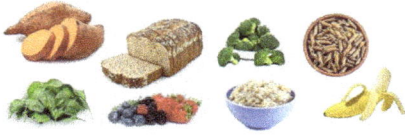

✘ SIMPLE CARBS

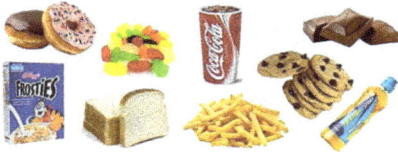

Macronutrients are the essential components of our diet that provide the energy and building blocks necessary for proper functioning of the body. Understanding macronutrients is fundamental to making informed dietary choices and achieving optimal health.

Let's explore one of the key macronutrients—carbohydrates, before getting into ingredients. We will discuss fats, proteins, and fiber later.

Carbohydrates serve as the body's primary source of energy and are vital for supporting various physiological functions. While simple carbohydrates provide quick energy boosts, complex carbohydrates offer sustained energy and essential nutrients crucial for overall health.

Prioritize complex carbohydrates found in whole grains, fruits, vegetables, and legumes, while limiting intake of added sugars. However, individualizing carbohydrate consumption is key, considering factors like activity level, health status, and personal goals.

It's worth noting that not all carbohydrates are inherently 'bad,' and low-carb diets may not be suitable for everyone. Each person's nutritional needs are unique, so it's essential to find a balanced approach that works best for you.

What simple carbs are you going to cut out?

Cut Simple Carbs

What about the ingredients?

Welcome to the Ingredients List section, where we will look at food additives, preservatives, and mysterious compounds lurking in our favorite snacks and meals. Get ready to uncover the secrets behind those unpronounceable names and discover why they're sprinkled, smothered, or injected into our foods.

So, grab your magnifying glass, and let's decode the cryptic language of food labels by looking at their purpose and their implications.

Less Concerning Ingredients

Ingredient Name	Purpose	Implications
Natural Flavors	Typically derived from natural sources such as fruits, vegetables, herbs, or spices to enhance the taste of food products.	Natural flavors are generally considered safe for consumption. However, it's essential to be aware that the term "natural flavors" can encompass a wide range of substances, including both naturally derived and synthetically produced compounds. While natural flavors are widely used in food products, individuals with specific allergies or sensitivities may need to exercise caution.
Sea Salt	A minimally processed form of salt that contains trace minerals and is often used as a flavor enhancer in foods.	Sea salt is a natural source of sodium and trace minerals, and it's often preferred over highly processed table salt. However, excessive consumption of sodium from any source can contribute to an individual's health issues.
Vinegar	Used as a preservative and flavoring agent in various foods, typically derived from fermented sources like wine, apples, or grains.	Vinegar is generally recognized as safe and has been used for centuries as a food preservative and flavor enhancer. It may offer potential health benefits, such as aiding digestion and regulating blood sugar levels. However, individuals with certain gastrointestinal conditions may need to limit their intake due to its acidity.
Citric Acid	A naturally occurring compound found in citrus fruits, often used as a flavoring agent, preservative, or acidity regulator in processed foods.	Citric acid is naturally found in citrus fruits and is widely used in the food industry as a flavoring agent, preservative, and acidity regulator. While it's generally regarded as safe, some individuals may experience adverse reactions, such as digestive discomfort, particularly when consumed in large quantities.

Less Concerning Ingredients, Cont.

Ingredient Name	Purpose	Implications
Xanthan Gum	A polysaccharide derived from fermented sugars, commonly used as a thickening agent and stabilizer in food products.	Xanthan gum is a commonly used food additive that is considered safe for consumption. It's well-tolerated by most individuals and is often used as a gluten-free alternative to thicken and stabilize food products. However, some people may experience gastrointestinal symptoms, such as bloating or gas, when consuming large amounts of xanthan gum.
Ascorbic Acid (Vitamin C)	A natural antioxidant and preservative found in fruits and vegetables, often added to food products to prevent oxidation and maintain color and freshness.	Ascorbic acid, or vitamin C, is an essential nutrient with antioxidant properties that plays a vital role in immune function, collagen synthesis, and wound healing. While it's generally safe for consumption, excessive intake may cause digestive upset or diarrhea in some individuals.
Tocopherols (Vitamin E)	Natural antioxidants derived from sources like soybean oil or wheat germ oil, used to prevent rancidity in fats and oils in processed foods.	Tocopherols, or vitamin E, are natural antioxidants commonly used in food products to prevent rancidity in fats and oils. They are generally regarded as safe and may offer potential health benefits, such as reducing oxidative stress and inflammation. However, excessive intake of vitamin E supplements may have adverse effects and should be avoided without medical supervision.
Honey	A natural sweetener produced by bees from flower nectar, often used as a flavoring agent and sweetener in various food products.	Honey is a natural sweetener produced by bees and is widely used in food products for its unique flavor and sweetness. It contains various nutrients and antioxidants, but it's also high in sugar and calories. While honey is generally safe for consumption, infants under one year of age should avoid consuming honey due to the risk of botulism.

Ingredient Name	Purpose	Implications
Herbs and Spices	Naturally occurring plant-based ingredients used to add flavor, aroma, and color to foods, with minimal processing and potential health benefits.	Herbs and spices are natural flavoring agents derived from plants and are rich in antioxidants, vitamins, and minerals. They can add depth of flavor and aroma to foods without adding extra calories, sodium, or fat. Incorporating herbs and spices into the diet can enhance the nutritional value of meals and contribute to overall health and well-being.
Whole Food Ingredients	Ingredients derived from whole, minimally processed foods such as fruits, vegetables, nuts, seeds, and whole grains, which provide essential nutrients and fiber without added chemicals or artificial additives.	Whole food ingredients, such as fruits, vegetables, nuts, seeds, and whole grains, are nutrient-dense and provide essential vitamins, minerals, fiber, and phytonutrients. Consuming a diet rich in whole foods can support overall health and reduce the risk of chronic diseases such as heart disease, diabetes, and obesity. Prioritizing whole foods over processed options is key to achieving optimal health and well-being.

Moderately Concerning Ingredients

Ingredient Name	Examples	Purpose	Implications
Emulsifiers	• Soy lecithin • Sunflower lecithin • Mono- and diglycerides • Polysorbate 80 • Polysorbate 60 • Glycerol monostearate • Sodium stearoyl lactylate • Carrageenan	Emulsifiers are used to stabilize and homogenize mixtures of liquids that would otherwise separate, such as oil and water. They help improve texture, consistency, and shelf life in a variety of processed foods, including baked goods, dressings, and ice cream.	Some studies suggest that certain emulsifiers may disrupt gut microbiota and contribute to intestinal inflammation in susceptible individuals.
Stabilizers and Thickeners	• Xanthan gum • Guar gum • Carrageenan • Cellulose gum • Pectin	Stabilizers and thickeners are used to enhance the texture, viscosity, and mouthfeel of food products. They help prevent separation, improve suspension of ingredients, and create a smoother, creamier texture in products like sauces, soups, and dairy alternatives.	Some individuals may experience digestive discomfort or allergic reactions to certain additives like carrageenan. There are concerns that carrageenan may contribute to intestinal inflammation and gastrointestinal symptoms in sensitive individuals.
Artificial Colors	• FD&C Red No. 40 (Allura Red AC) • FD&C Yellow No. 5 (Tartrazine) • FD&C Yellow No. 6 (Sunset Yellow FCF) • FD&C Blue No. 1 (Brilliant Blue FCF) • FD&C Green No. 3 (Fast Green FCF)	Artificial colors are added to foods and beverages to enhance their visual appeal, create distinctive colors, and make products more attractive to consumers. They are commonly used in a wide range of processed foods, including candies, sodas, and packaged snacks.	Artificial colors have been linked to hyperactivity and behavioral issues in children, although the evidence is mixed. Some individuals may also experience allergic reactions or intolerance to certain artificial colors. Additionally, some artificial colors have been associated with cancer.

Ingredient Name	Examples	Purpose	Implications
Artificial Flavors	• ethylvanillin • ethyl methylphenyl-glycidate • methyl anthranilate • gamma-decalactone	Artificial flavors are synthetic compounds designed to mimic natural flavors and enhance the taste and aroma of food products. They are often used to create specific flavor profiles or mask undesirable tastes in processed foods, such as confectionery, desserts, and savory snacks.	Some individuals may have sensitivities or allergies to certain synthetic compounds. Additionally, reliance on artificial flavors may contribute to a disconnection from natural flavors and whole foods, potentially impacting taste preferences and dietary choices.
Preservatives	• Sodium benzoate • Potassium sorbate • Calcium propionate • Sodium nitrite • BHA (Butylated hydroxyanisole)	Preservatives are added to foods to prevent spoilage, inhibit microbial growth, and extend shelf life. They help maintain the freshness, quality, and safety of processed foods by inhibiting oxidation, mold, and bacterial contamination.	Some preservatives, such as BHA and BHT, have been classified as possible carcinogens by regulatory agencies. While they are permitted for use in food products at low levels, there are concerns about their potential long-term health effects, including carcinogenicity and endocrine disruption.
MSG	Monosodium Glutamate	MSG is a flavor enhancer used to enhance the savory taste of foods, often referred to as umami. It is commonly used in savory snacks, canned soups, and Asian cuisine to boost flavor perception and improve overall taste satisfaction.	MSG has been associated with the phenomenon known as "Chinese Restaurant Syndrome," characterized by symptoms such as headache, nausea, and chest tightness in some individuals.

Highly Concerning Ingredients

Ingredient Name	Examples	Purpose	Implications
Artificial Sweeteners	• Aspartame • Sucralose • Saccharin • Acesulfame potassium (Ace-K) • Neotame	Artificial sweeteners are often used as sugar substitutes to provide sweetness without the calories or carbohydrates of sugar. They are commonly found in "diet" or "sugar-free" products to reduce calorie content and appeal to consumers looking to limit their sugar intake.	Artificial sweeteners have been the subject of controversy regarding their safety and potential health effects. While they are approved for use by regulatory agencies, some studies suggest that artificial sweeteners may be associated with adverse metabolic effects, such as weight gain, altered gut microbiota, and increased cravings for sweet foods. Additionally, there are concerns about their potential impact on insulin sensitivity and blood sugar regulation, although research findings are mixed.
Hydrogenated Oils (AKA Trans Fats)	• Hydrogenated soybean oil, cottonseed oil, palm oil, or coconut oil • Partially hydrogenated vegetable oil, or palm kernel oil	Hydrogenated oils are used to solidify liquid oils and extend the shelf life of processed foods. They are commonly found in margarine, shortening, baked goods, fried foods, and snack products to improve texture, flavor, and stability.	Hydrogenated oils contain trans fats, which are known to increase levels of LDL (bad) cholesterol and lower levels of HDL (good) cholesterol, thereby increasing the risk of cardiovascular disease. Consumption of trans fats has been linked to coronary heart disease, stroke, and other adverse health outcomes. In addition, hydrogenated oils may also contribute to inflammation and oxidative stress in the body, further increasing the risk of chronic diseases.
High-Fructose Corn Syrup (HFCS)	Made from corn, but we will discuss the process later.	High-fructose corn syrup is a sweetener derived from corn starch and is used as a cheaper alternative to sucrose (table sugar) in many processed foods and beverages. It provides sweetness, enhances flavor, and improves texture in a wide range of products, including soft drinks, baked goods, and processed snacks.	High-fructose corn syrup has been linked to various health issues, including obesity, insulin resistance, type 2 diabetes, fatty liver disease, and metabolic syndrome. HFCS is metabolized differently in the body compared to sucrose (table sugar), leading to elevated levels of triglycerides and uric acid, which can contribute to insulin resistance and metabolic dysfunction. Excessive consumption of HFCS, particularly in the form of sugary beverages and processed foods, may significantly increase the risk of developing these chronic conditions.

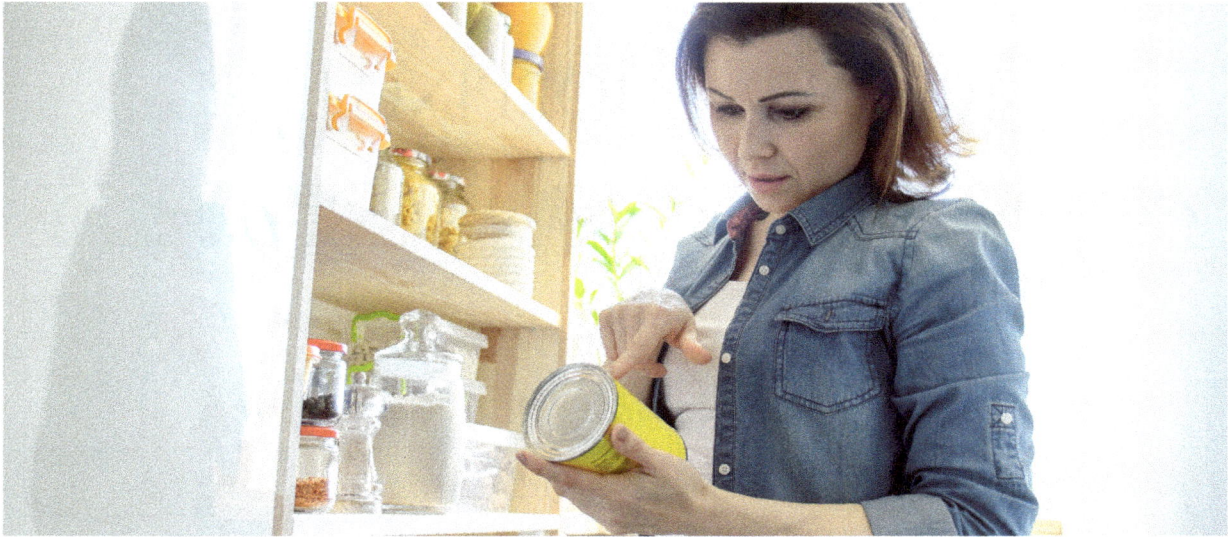

Action Steps

1

Go through your pantry and read the labels. How many processed foods do you currently have? How much sugar is in your food and condiments?

2

Consider removing some of them from your home and replace with whole foods.

3

Make a new grocery list of all the whole foods you want to start incorporating into your diet.

_____

_____

_____

GROCERY SHOPPING LIST

✓	MEAT / FISH / DAIRY	QTY

✓	FRUITS & VEGETABLES	QTY

✓	PANTRY ITEMS	QTY

✓	FREEZER ITEMS	QTY

✓	NUTS & SEEDS	QTY

✓	MISCELLANEOS	QTY

New Start

What are some
of the foods that
you will
permanently
remove from
your diet?

Start Healing

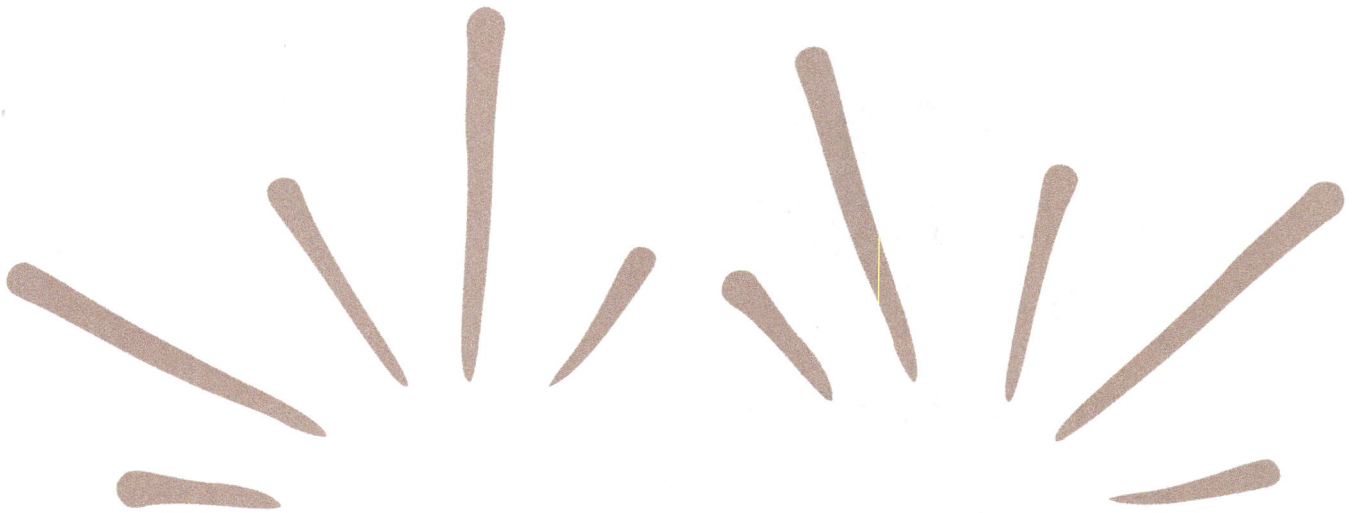

Remember to always
go slowly when making
dietary changes.

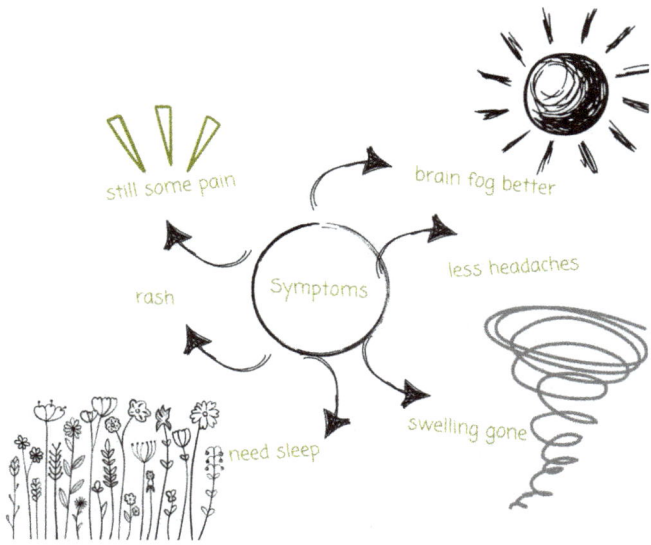

Track It!

Feel free to use the lines on this page to jot down your symptoms, mood, or anything else that comes to mind— or you could even doodle it!

still some pain

brain fog better

rash

Symptoms

less headaches

need sleep

swelling gone

Track It

Reflection Time

Change can be difficult, but I believe you can do it. Take baby steps. It doesn't have to be done in one day. How will you implement these changes?

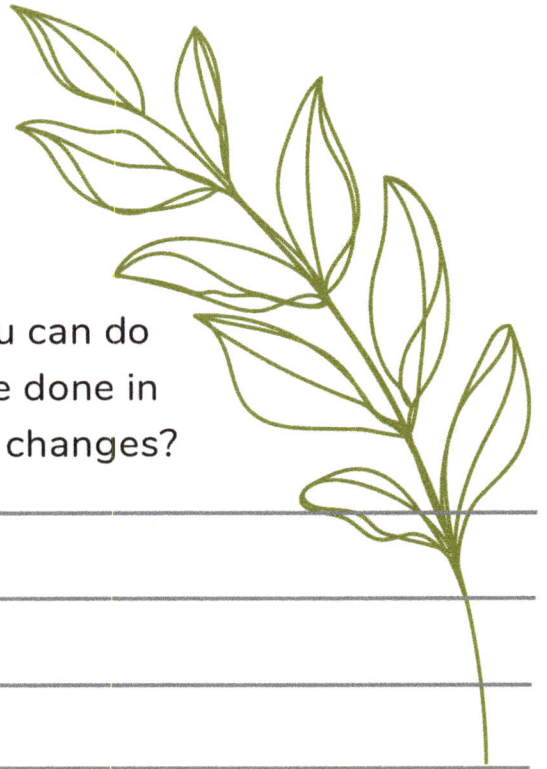

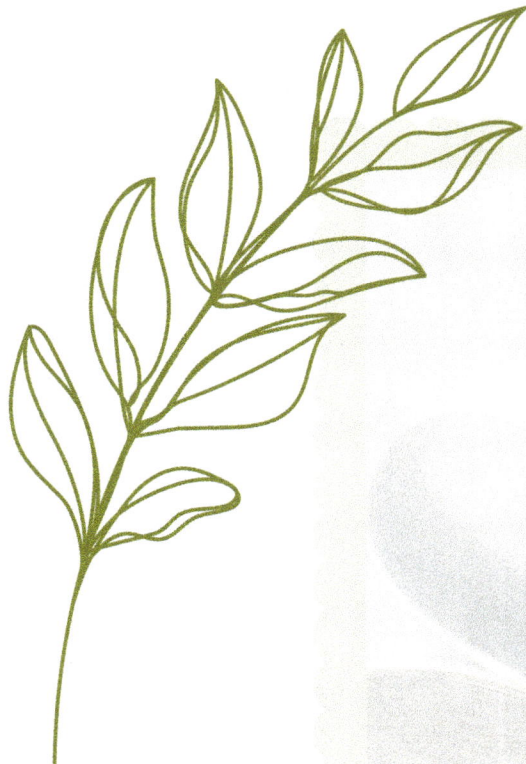

_____

_____

_____

_____

Isaiah 43:19

See, I am doing a new thing! Now it springs up; do you not perceive it? I am making a way in the wilderness and streams in the wasteland

God's Word

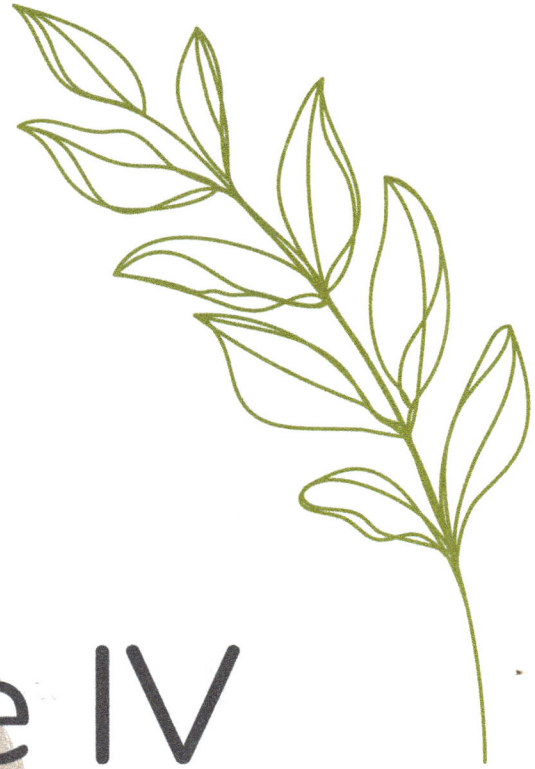

Phase IV

Sleep

DO NOT DISTURB

Thank You

How is your sleep?

SLEEP HISTORY

SELECT THE BEST RATING SCALE FOR EACH STATEMENT.

Statement	Rating Scale			
	Never	Monthly	Weekly	Daily
I struggle to fall asleep within 20 minutes of going to bed.	○	○	○	○
I wake up during the night and find it hard to fall back asleep.	○	○	○	○
I wake up feeling tired or not well-rested.	○	○	○	○
I feel sleepy or sluggish during the day.	○	○	○	○
I rely on sleep aids (medication or supplements) to help me sleep.	○	○	○	○
I wake up multiple times during the night.	○	○	○	○
I feel anxious or restless when trying to fall asleep.	○	○	○	○

IF YOU ANSWERED ANYTHING OTHER THAN 'NEVER', IT'S TIME TO WORK ON IMPROVING YOUR SLEEP!

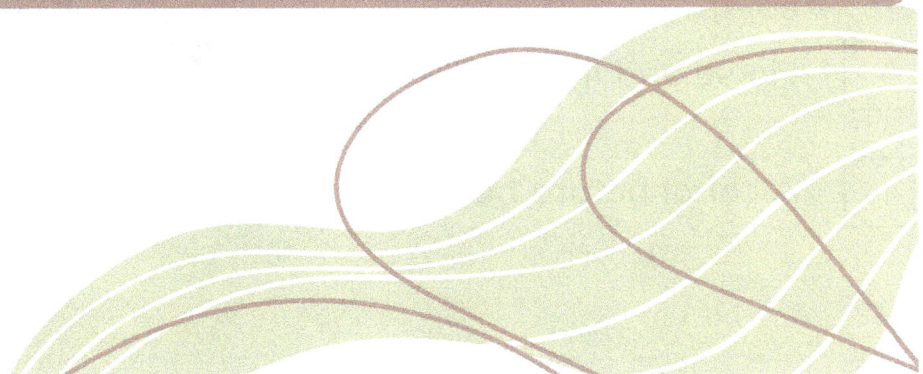

Sleep Stealers

Consistently poor sleep can contribute to undiagnosed health problems, like chronic fatigue, brain fog, hormone imbalances, digestive issues, and increased sensitivity to stress. Over time, lack of quality rest can quietly disrupt your body's ability to function at its best, often without obvious symptoms at first. What are your sleep stealers?

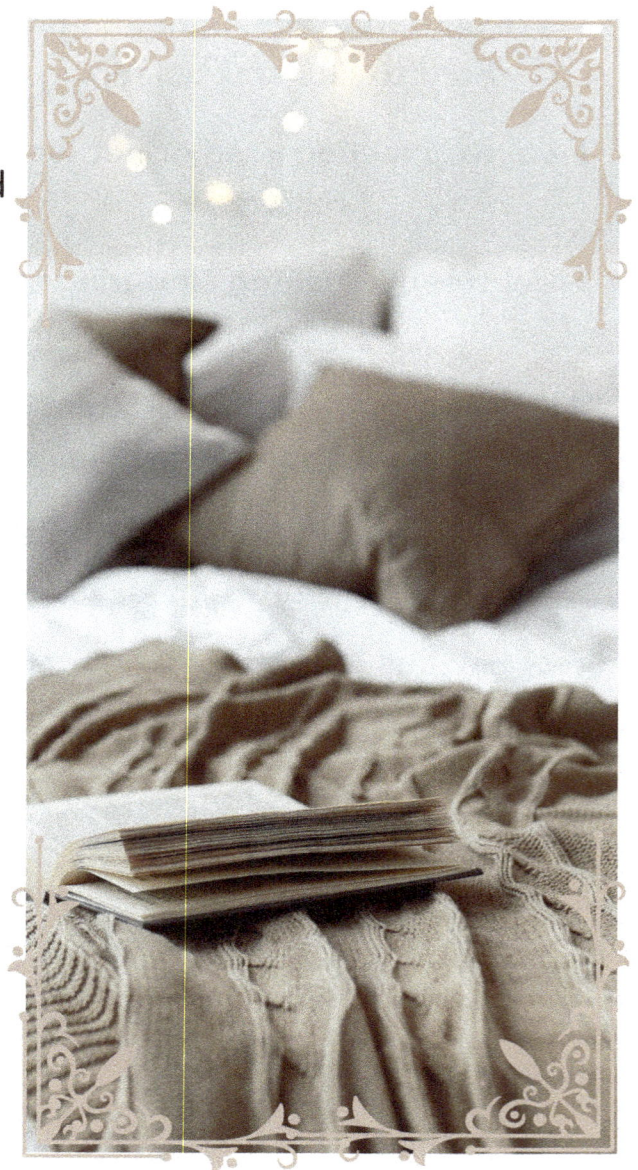

- ☐ TV in bedroom

- ☐ Use of electronics before bed

- ☐ Stress and anxiety

- ☐ Caffeine and sugar

- ☐ Irregular sleep schedule

- ☐ Eating large, late meals

- ☐ Lack of bedtime routine

- ☐ Room temperature (hot or cold)

- ☐ Noise and light pollution

- ☐ Alcohol before bed

Evaluate your sleep space. What are you going to change?

More Details...

IMPORTANCE OF SLEEP

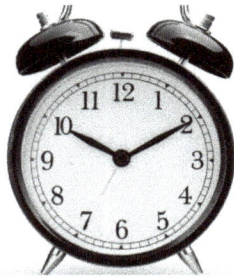

Sufficient sleep is non-negotiable. Poor sleep not only disrupts hormonal balance, including insulin regulation, but it can also contribute to heightened inflammation in the body. Aim for 7-9 hours of quality sleep per night to support overall health, regulate blood sugar, and minimize inflammation.

Section 1: The Melatonin Cycle of Circadian Rhythm

Melatonin, the sleep hormone, plays a pivotal role in our circadian rhythms (body's internal clock).

• Light exposure, suppresses melatonin release, signaling wakefulness.

• Darkness stimulates the pineal gland to produce and release melatonin, promoting restful sleep and maintaining circadian balance.

Circadian rhythm in healthy individuals

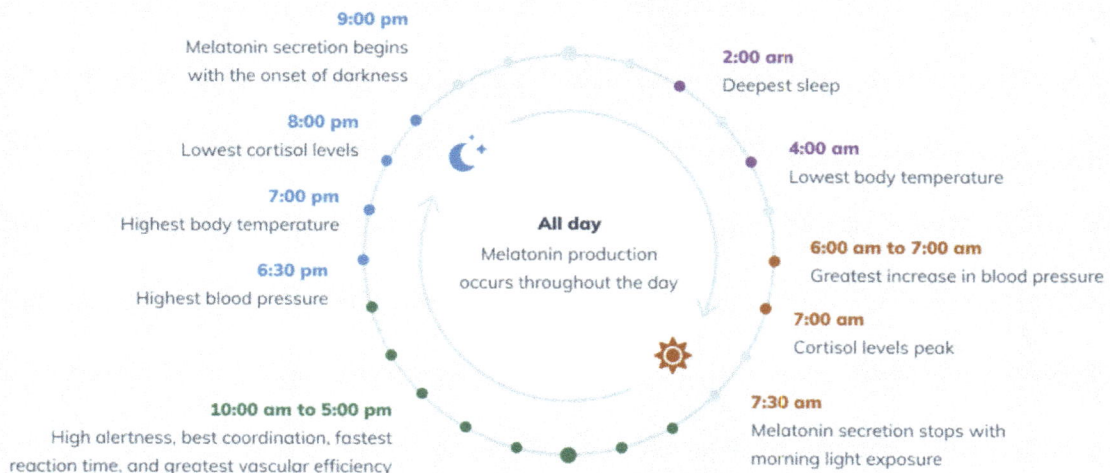

9:00 pm
Melatonin secretion begins with the onset of darkness

2:00 am
Deepest sleep

8:00 pm
Lowest cortisol levels

4:00 am
Lowest body temperature

7:00 pm
Highest body temperature

All day
Melatonin production occurs throughout the day

6:00 am to 7:00 am
Greatest increase in blood pressure

6:30 pm
Highest blood pressure

7:00 am
Cortisol levels peak

10:00 am to 5:00 pm
High alertness, best coordination, fastest reaction time, and greatest vascular efficiency

7:30 am
Melatonin secretion stops with morning light exposure

Section 2: Creating the Ideal Sleep Environment

Eliminate sources of light by:
- covering up glowing lights, such as those from the TV.
- removing devices like smartphones, tablets, and computers or maintaining a 5-foot radius free from plugs and devices.

Establish a consistent sleep schedule:
- Go to bed and wake up at the same time every day, even on weekends. This helps regulate your body's internal clock.

Create a relaxing bedtime routine:
- Develop pre-sleep rituals like reading a book, taking a warm bath, or practicing relaxation exercises to signal to your body that it's time to wind down.

Get regular exercise:
- Engage in regular physical activity but try to finish exercising at least a few hours before bedtime.

Manage stress:
- Practice stress-reducing techniques such as deep breathing, meditation, or yoga to help calm the mind before bedtime.

These simple changes contribute to an optimal sleep environment.

Creating an **optimal sleep environment**

Limit light exposure

Use curtains or blinds to block exterior light, and unplug light-emitting devices.

Keep electronics out of the bedroom

Keep your phone out of reach, and don't keep a TV in your bedroom.

Set your thermostat to a comfortable temperature

68 to 72°F (20 to 22°C) is believed to be the most ideal temperature range for sleep.

Eliminate unwanted noises

Keep windows closed, and use ear plugs to avoid exposure to noise.

Opt for a medium-firm mattress

Studies show that a medium-firm mattress is the best option for promoting sleep quality and comfort.

Choose the right pillow for you

The type of pillow that's right for you largely depends on your personal preferences and sleep position.

Consider essential oils

Add a few drops of a relaxing essential oil such as lavender or chamomile to a diffuser.

Encourage pets to sleep in their own beds

Bed sharing with pets can disrupt the quality of your sleep.

Section 3: Natural Boosters for Melatonin Production

Avoiding substances that inhibit melatonin is essential. Substances that can interfere are:

- NSAIDs
- large doses of vitamin B-12
- caffeine
- steroids
- alcohol

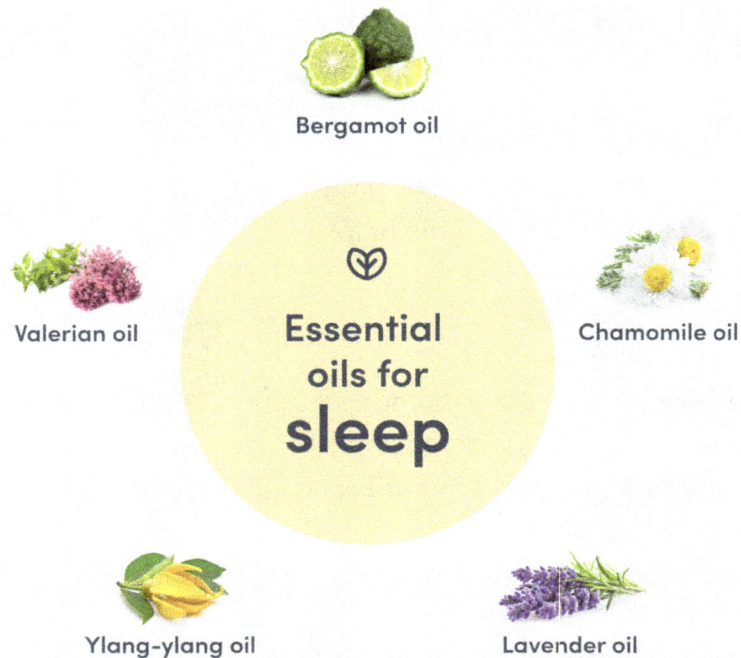

Essential oils for **sleep**

Bergamot oil

Chamomile oil

Lavender oil

Ylang-ylang oil

Valerian oil

Instead, explore natural options like:

- purslane, a leafy green with high melatonin levels.
- tryptophan-rich foods like turkey or pumpkin seeds.
- Montmorency cherry juice.
- essential oils

Sweet dreams await when you prioritize melatonin and embrace a holistic approach to sleep.

STRESS MANAGEMENT TECHNIQUES

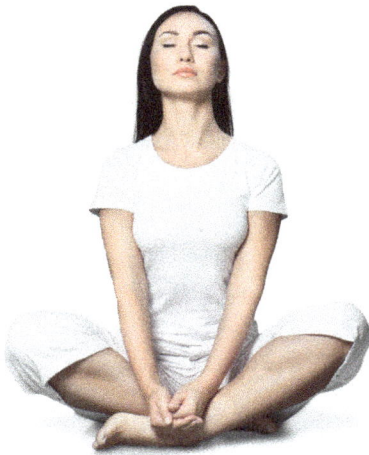

Stress is the way our body and mind react to pressure, challenges, or difficult situations. When confronted with a stressor, whether real or imagined, the body activates the "fight-or-flight" response, releasing stress hormones such as cortisol and adrenaline.

Physiological changes during stress include increased heart rate, elevated blood pressure, heightened alertness, and energy mobilization. These changes are designed to help the body respond quickly to a threat. In the short term, stress can be beneficial, improving focus and performance.

However, chronic or excessive stress can have negative effects on physical and mental health. Prolonged exposure to stress hormones can contribute to various health issues, including cardiovascular problems, immune system suppression, digestive disorders, and mental health conditions such as anxiety and depression.

Effective stress management involves recognizing stressors, implementing coping strategies, and maintaining a healthy balance in life to minimize the negative impact of stress.

Here are some practical tips to help alleviate stress:

Deep Breathing:
1

Practice deep breathing exercises to calm your nervous system. Inhale slowly through your nose, hold for a few seconds and exhale through your mouth.

Mindfulness Meditation:
2

Engage in mindfulness meditation to focus on the present moment. This can help break the cycle of worry and anxiety.

Regular Exercise:
3

Physical activity is a natural stress reliever. Incorporate regular exercise into your routine, whether it's walking, jogging, yoga, or any activity you enjoy.

Adequate Sleep:
4

Ensure you get enough quality sleep each night. Lack of sleep can contribute to increased stress levels.

Healthy Diet:
5

Eat a balanced diet rich in whole foods. Nutrient-dense foods can positively impact mood and energy levels.

6

Time Management:
Organize your tasks and prioritize effectively. Break down large tasks into smaller, manageable steps.

7

Social Support:
Maintain connections with friends and family. Sharing your feelings with others can provide emotional support.

8

Hobbies and Relaxation:
Engage in activities you enjoy, whether it's reading, listening to music, or spending time in nature. This can provide a mental break and promote relaxation.

9

Limit Stimulants:
Reduce your intake of caffeine and other stimulants, especially in the evening, to support better sleep.

10

Seek Professional Help:
If stress becomes overwhelming, consider seeking support from a mental health professional.

Track It!

Feel free to use the lines on this page to jot down your symptoms, mood, or anything else that comes to mind— or you could even doodle it!

still some pain

brain fog better

rash

Symptoms

less headaches

need sleep

swelling gone

Track It

Reflection Time

Start taking small steps to help you with your sleep. What will you start with?

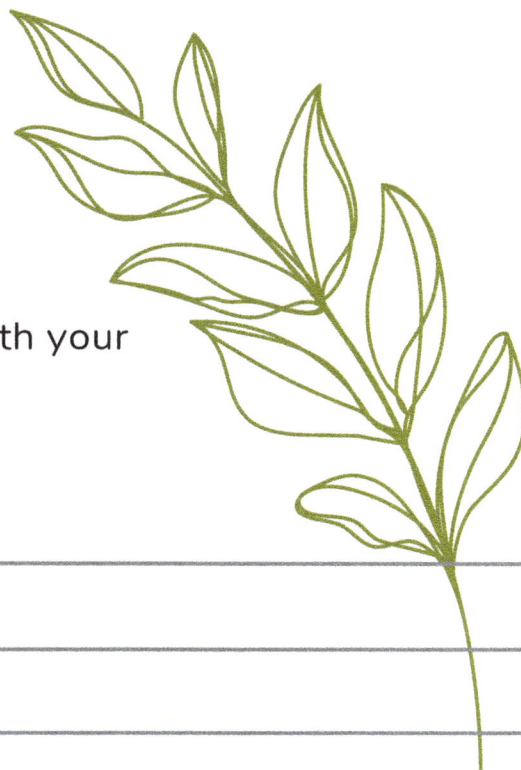

_____

_____

_____

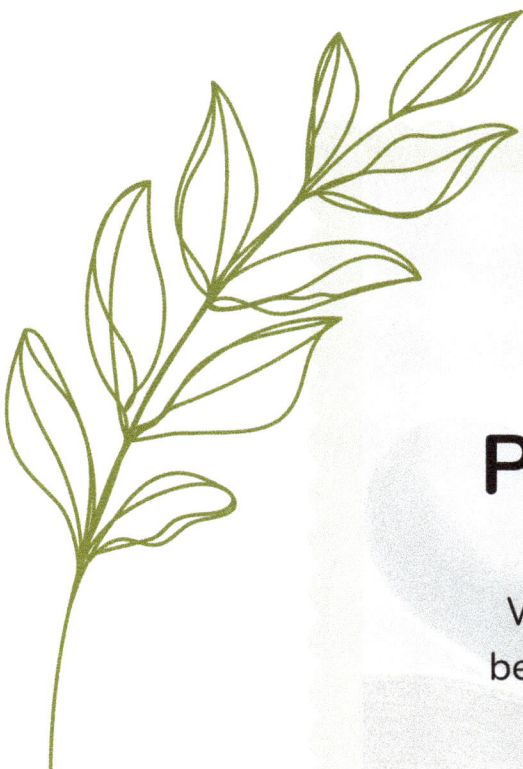

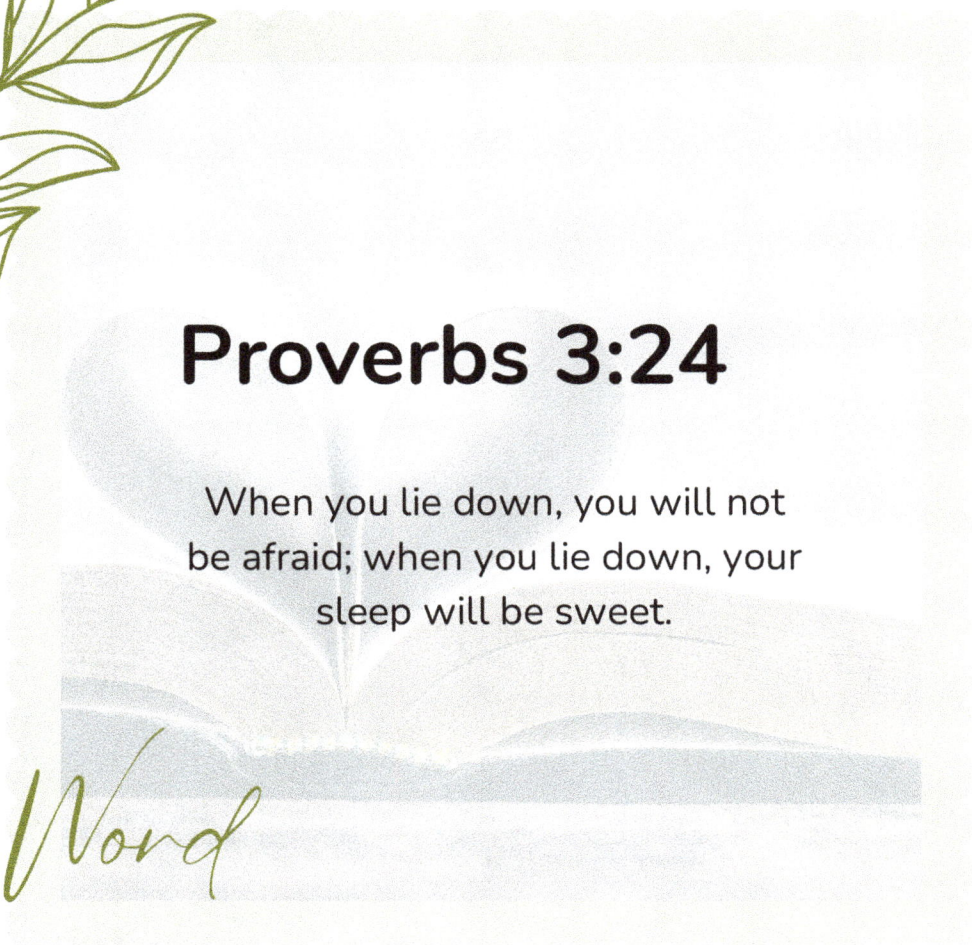

Proverbs 3:24

When you lie down, you will not be afraid; when you lie down, your sleep will be sweet.

God's Word

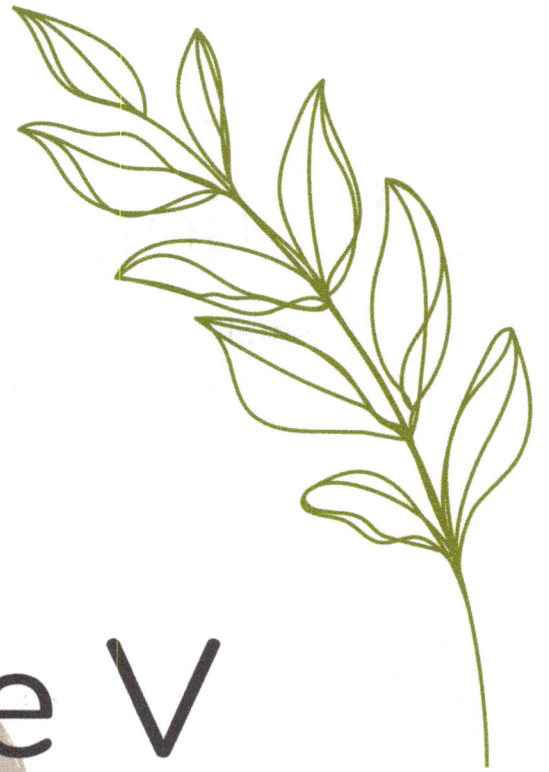

Phase V

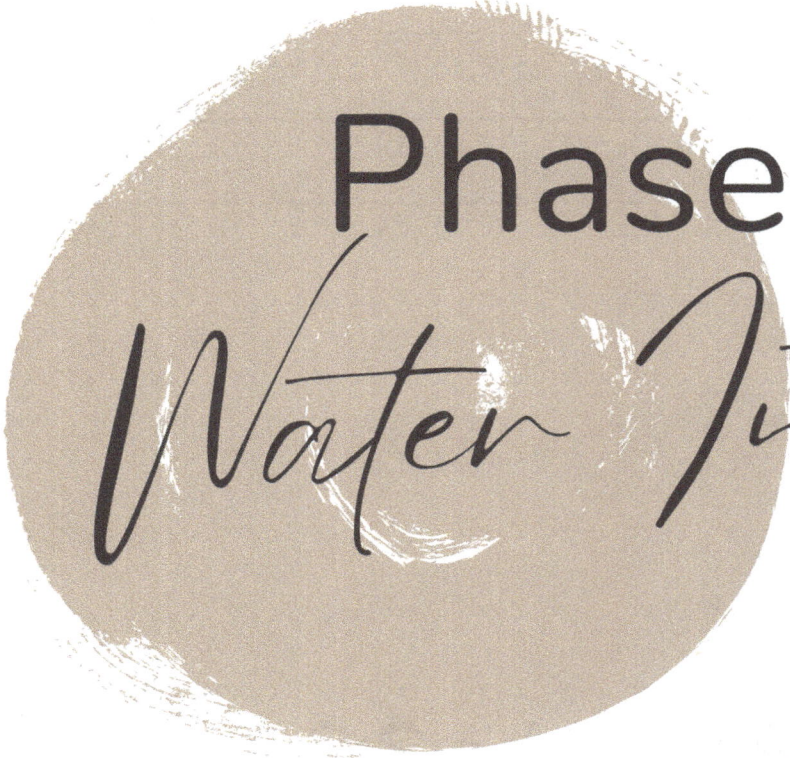
Water Intake

dizziness

headaches

fevers   chills

dry skin   rapid heartbeat

Dehydration can cause symptoms common with undiagnosed illnesses.

sunken eyes   brain fog

fatigue

dark-colored urine

dry mouth & lips

Did you know?

Several markers on your bloodwork give us a clue that you are dehydrated. If any of the following are elevated on your bloodwork, it could indicate dehydration:

- Red Blood Cell (RBC)
- Blood Urea Nitrogen (BUN)
- Sodium
- Potassium
- Chloride
- Protein
- Albumin

GENERAL HEALTH	Result
White Blood Cell Count Desired Range: 3.8-10.8 Thousand/uL	5.9
Red Blood Cell Count Desired Range: 3.80-5.10 Million/uL	4.44
Hemoglobin Desired Range: 11.7-15.5 g/dL	13.0
Hematocrit Desired Range: 35.0-45.0 %	40.3
Mean RBC Volume Desired Range: 80.0-100.0 fL	90.8
Mean RBC Iron Desired Range: 27.0-33.0 pg	29.3
Mean RBC Iron Concentration Desired Range: 32.0-36.0 g/dL	32.3
RBC Distribution Width Desired Range: 11.0-15.0 %	12.8
Platelets Desired Range: 140-400 Thousand/uL	300
MPV Desired Range: 7.5-12.5 fL	10.8
Absolute Neutrophils Desired Range: 1500-7800 cells/uL	3404
Absolute Lymphocytes Desired Range: 850-3900 cells/uL	1811
Absolute Monocytes Desired Range: 200-950 cells/uL	502

Of course, there are several other reasons these could be high and should not be taken lightly if they are.

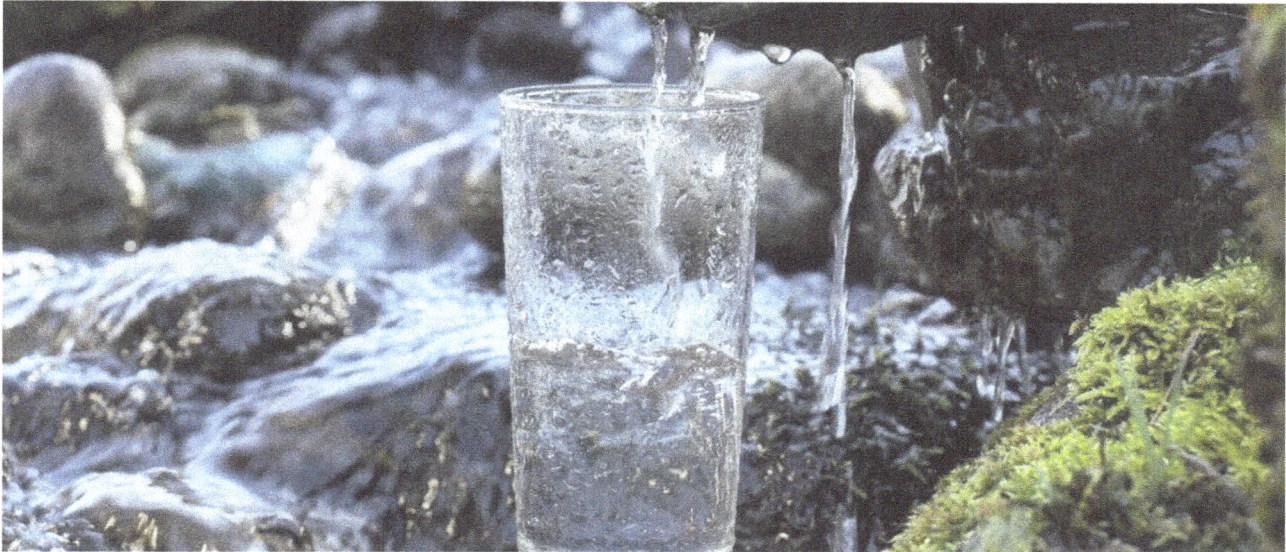

Action Steps

1

2

3

Calculate personal water intake goal.

Increase your water intake as needed. Try the 10 tips on the following pages.

Track your water intake and track how you are feeling!

To calculate your personal water intake goal:

- Multiply your body weight (in pounds) by 0.5 to find the number of ounces you should drink each day.

- Example: For a 150-pound person: 150 x 0.5 = 75 ounces per day.

More Details...
DRINK YOUR WATER - 10 TIPS

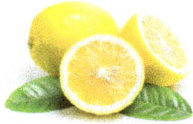

Lemon Love - Add lemon or lime slices to dress it up and support your body's detox pathways.

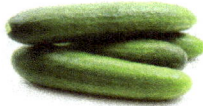

Eat Your Veggies - Slip in some veggies and fruits that pack a hydrating punch like celery, cucumber, watermelon, and cantaloupe.

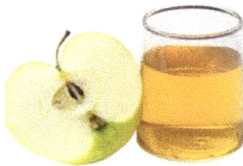

Brain Tonic - Make a morning "tonic" with apple cider vinegar and adaptogenic tinctures like schizandra, ashwagandha, or rhodiola.

Morning Ritual - Make a large glass of water part of your daily routine by having your water bottle next to your sink ready to drink before you even brush your teeth.

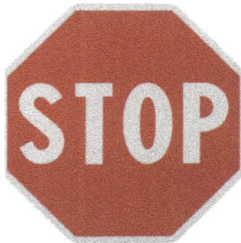

Drink and Drive - Keep a water bottle in your car and sip while you're stopped in traffic or waiting in the carpool line.

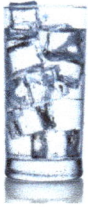

Curb Your Cravings - When sweet cravings strike, have a glass of water before you turn to the chocolate (you might be dehydrated and not hungry!)

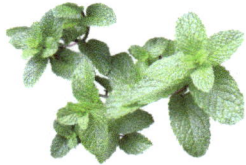

Get Herby - Create a unique taste by adding freshly muddled herbs to your water; try fresh peppermint, lemongrass, lavender, or cilantro.

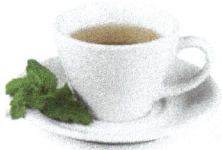

Tea Party - Hot or iced, adding more herbal teas to your day increases your water intake and nutrition.

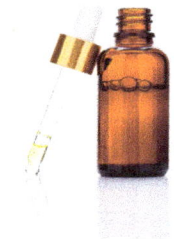

Oil and Water - Add a drop or two of essential oil to boost the flavor of your water; peppermint, orange, and lavender all make water taste delicious. (Just be sure to use oils that are safe for consumption.)

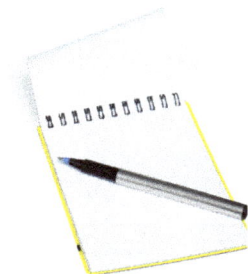

Track It - Shine a light on how much you are actually drinking by tracking for five days – no judgment, just be curious and get clear on how you can drink more water.

DAILY WATER INTAKE

WEEK ....   DAILY GOAL ....   RESULT ....

SUNDAY
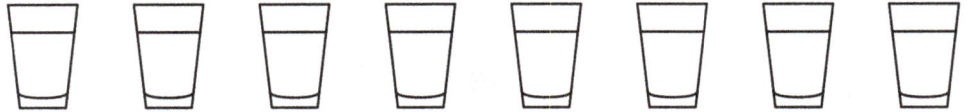

MONDAY
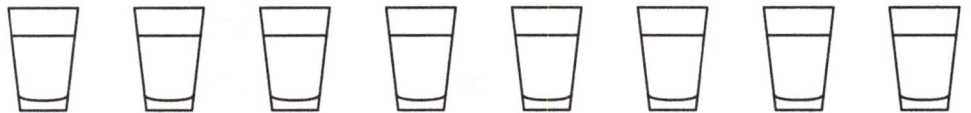

TUESDAY
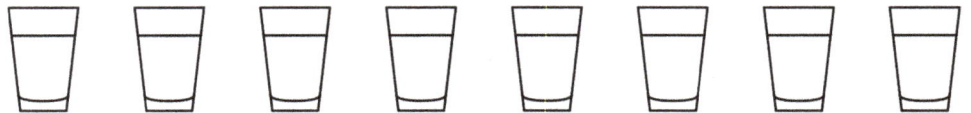

WEDNESDAY
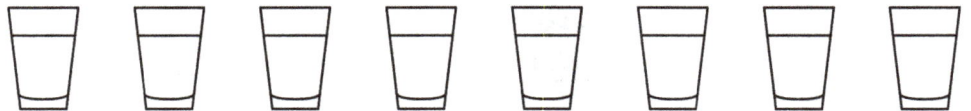

THURSDAY
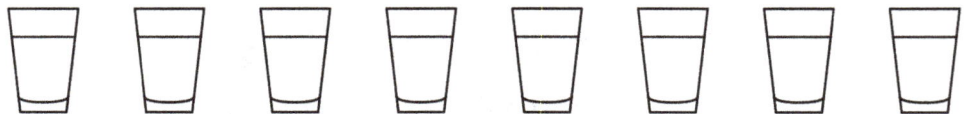

FRIDAY
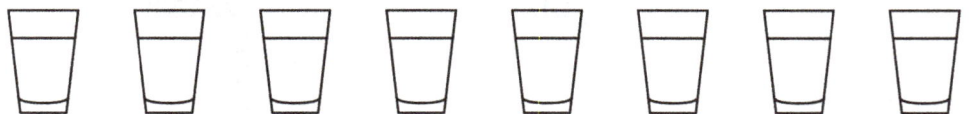

SATURDAY
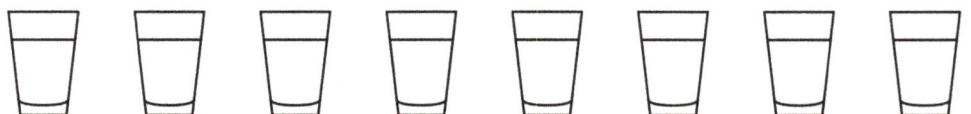

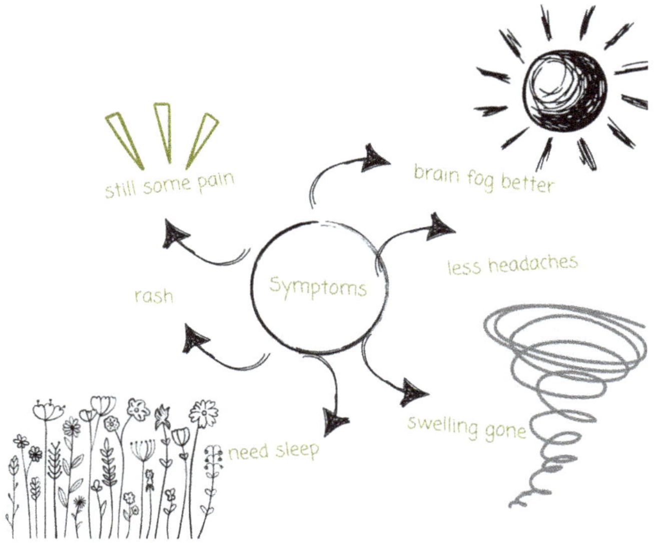

Track It!

Feel free to use the lines on this page to jot down your symptoms, mood, or anything else that comes to mind— or you could even doodle it!

still some pain

brain fog better

rash

Symptoms

less headaches

need sleep

swelling gone

Track It

Reflection Time

Did you know that God designed our bodies to be made up of approximately 60% water?

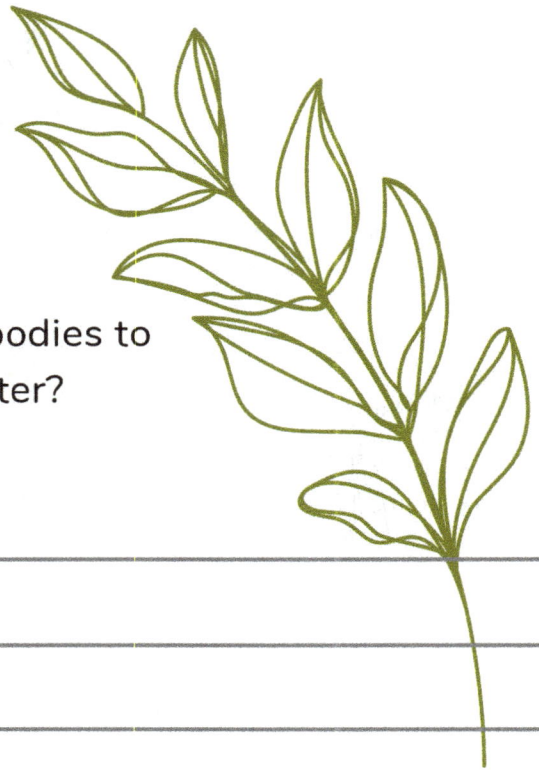

_____

_____

_____

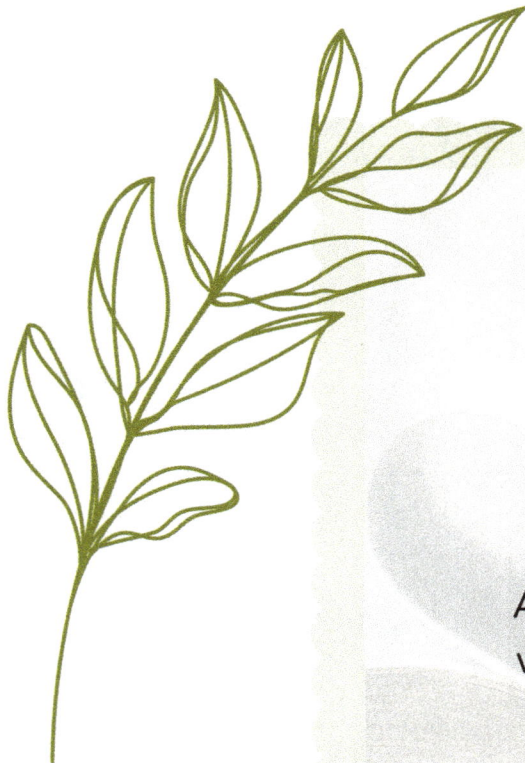

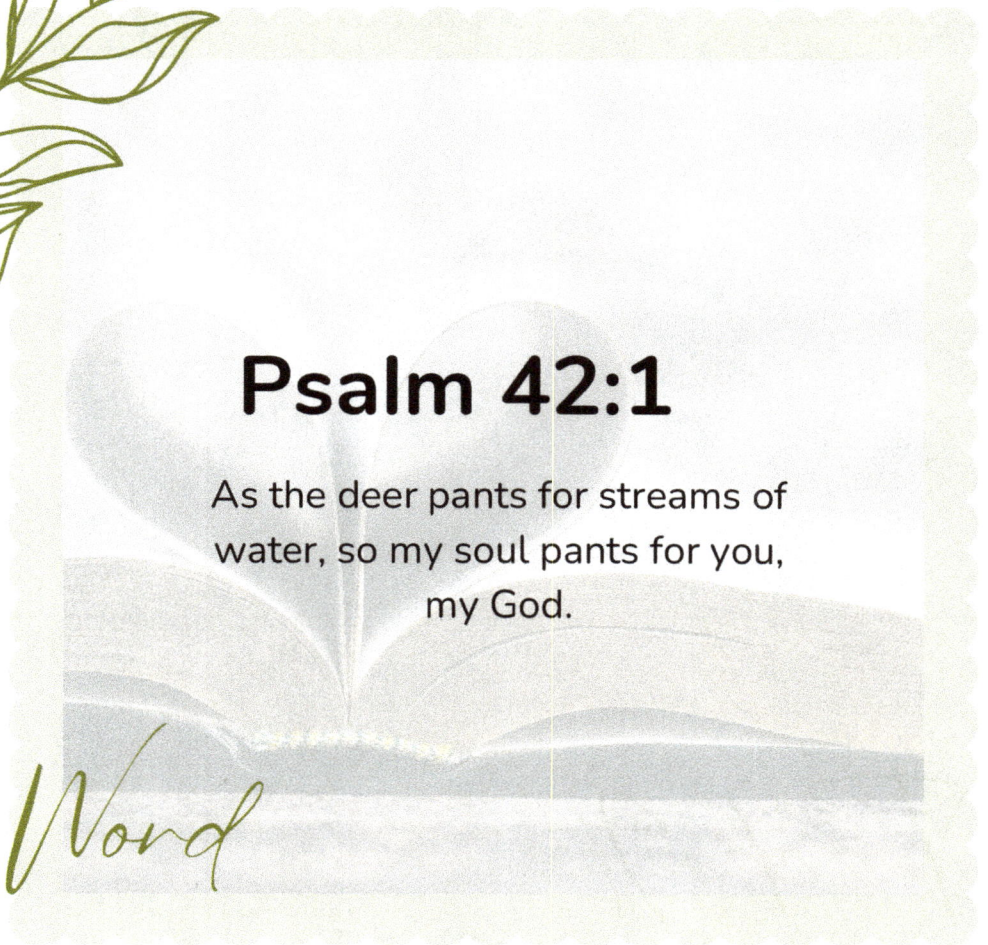

Psalm 42:1

As the deer pants for streams of water, so my soul pants for you, my God.

God's Word

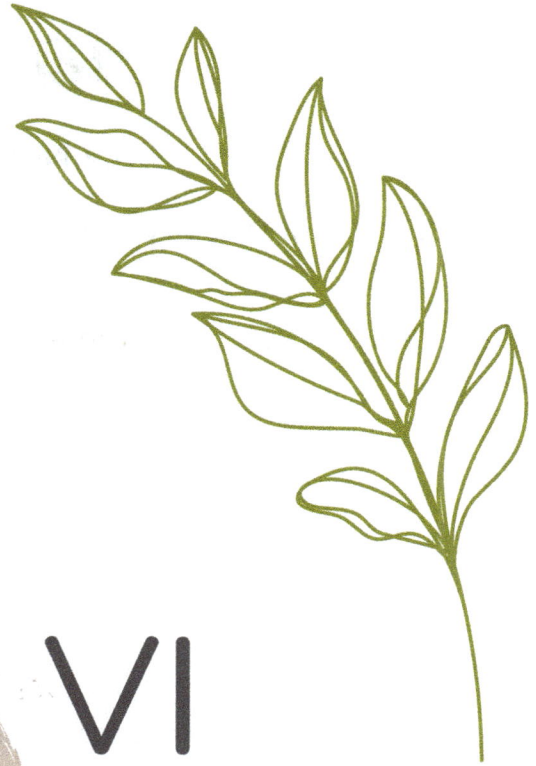

Phase VI

Take it up a Notch

How Have You Done?

Before we "Take it up a Notch", let's reflect on how you've done so far.

Document the results of your efforts.

- Removed inflammatory foods:

- Replaced with whole foods and anti-inflammatory foods:

- Improved sleep habits:

- Increased water intake:

NOURISH YOUR BODY

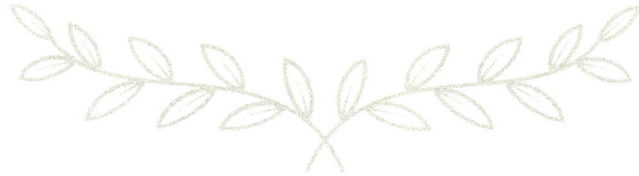

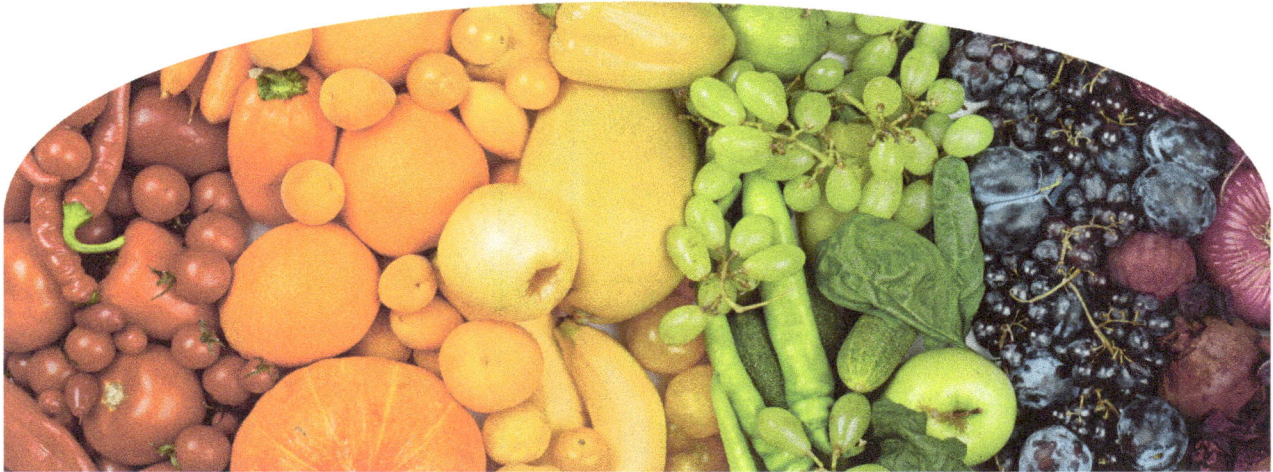

EAT THE RAINBOW

To give our bodies all the nutrients and vitamins they need, it is important to eat a variety of foods in a variety of colors.

Each color of food provides different vitamins and nutrients.

Let's see how well you are currently doing.

Nourishment

Current Nutrition Intake:

MONDAY

TUESDAY

WEDNESDAY

THURSDAY

FRIDAY

SATURDAY

SUNDAY

Rainbow

Directions:

Jot down what you eat daily.

At the end of the week, check off the colors of **fruits** and **vegetables** that you ate.

No, Skittles do not count!

Colors:

○ Red
○ Yellow
○ Orange
○ Green
○ Purple
○ Blue
○ White

With this new information, what new foods will you try this week?

More Details...

EAT FOR HEALTH

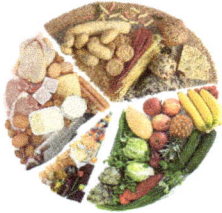

In functional nutrition, we recognize that everyone is unique; what works for one, may not work for another. Below are general Eat for Health suggestions. As you make changes, see how you feel and then make adjustments accordingly. This is why we track everything!

- Focus on whole foods, particularly high protein foods with high nutrient density at each meal.

- Eat grass-fed beef, pastured chicken, and low-mercury, fresh seafood (not farmed) whenever possible to reduce exposure to pesticides and toxins.

- Eat 3 meals a day plus snacks to maintain blood sugar.

- Eat organic pastured eggs, at least one per day.

- Minimize soy intake with the exception of fermented soy in the form of miso, tempeh, and shoyu with non-GMO tofu and edamame on occasion.

- Eliminate refined wheat.

- Incorporate non-glutinous grains, such as brown rice, quinoa, millet, amaranth, and buckwheat.

- Include healthy fats such as:
  - coconut oil and ghee for cooking.
  - cold press extra virgin olive oil, flax, and hemp oil for salad dressing (flax and hemp are never to be heated; olive oil is never used with high heat).
  - sesame, sunflower, and pumpkin are all good seed choices.
  - avocado and olives into your diet with regularity.
  - nuts and seeds in their raw or sprouted form - the latter will ease digestion - and in the form of nut butters (minimize peanuts and peanut butter)

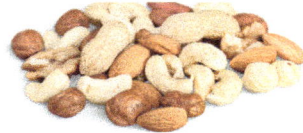

- Include as many fermented foods in the diet as possible.
  - Yogurt
  - Sauerkraut
  - Kimchi
  - Kombucha
  - Miso
  - Tempeh
  - Pickles
  - Fermented Cheese: Certain types of cheese, like Gouda or cheddar, go through a fermentation process.

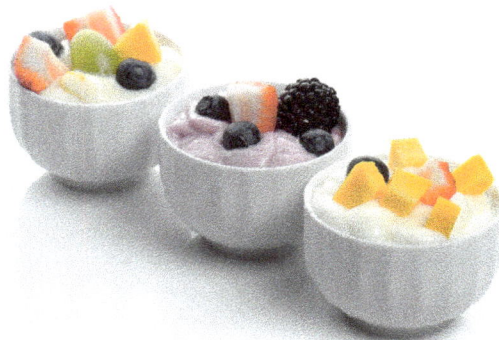

New Nutrition Intake:

MONDAY

TUESDAY

WEDNESDAY

THURSDAY

FRIDAY

SATURDAY

SUNDAY

Rainbow

Directions:

Jot down what you eat daily.

At the end of the week, check off the colors of **fruits** and **vegetables** that you ate.

Colors:

- ○ Red
- ○ Yellow
- ○ Orange
- ○ Green
- ○ Purple
- ○ Blue
- ○ White

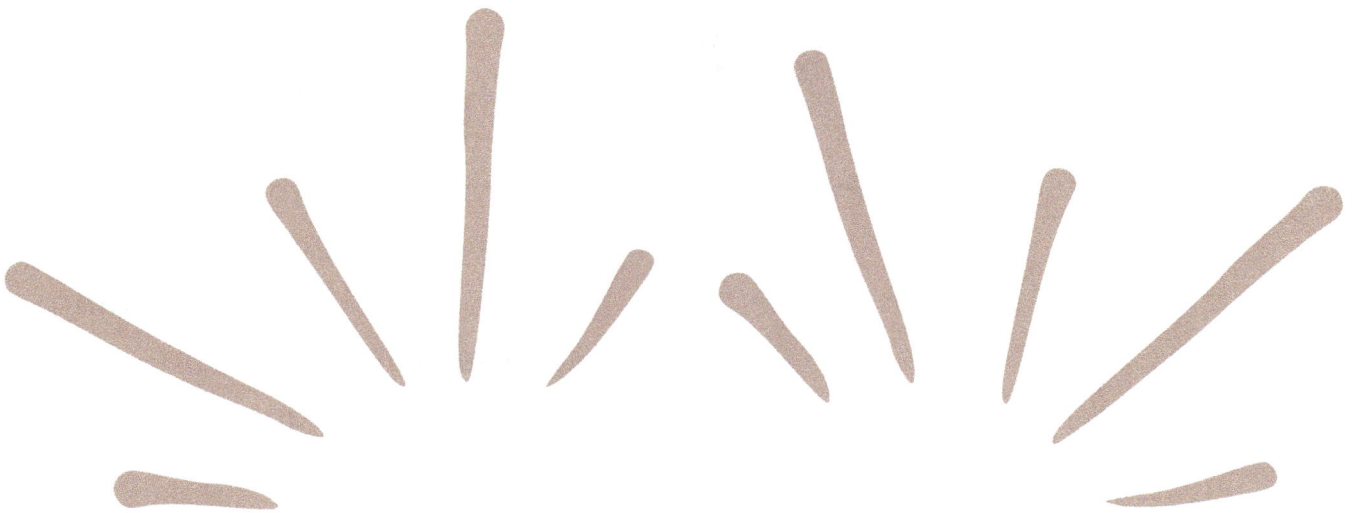

Remember to always
go slowly when making
dietary changes.

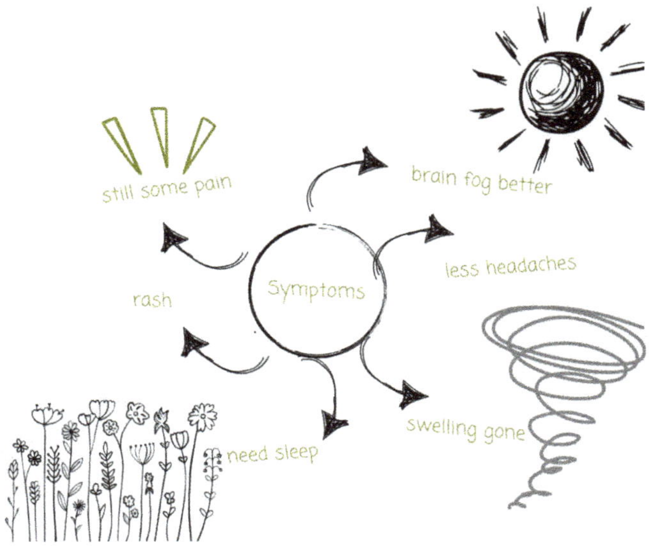

still some pain

brain fog better

rash

Symptoms

less headaches

need sleep

swelling gone

Track It!

Feel free to use the lines on this page to jot down your symptoms, mood, or anything else that comes to mind— or you could even doodle it!

Track It

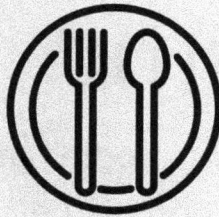

HEALTHY EATING

"

EATING HEALTHY SHOULD NOT FEEL LIKE A DIET. IT SHOULD FEEL LIKE YOU ARE FINALLY EATING!

"

S. H.

Reflection Time

God created food to nourish our bodies and help us thrive. Choosing the right foods is key to experiencing the fullness of His provision.

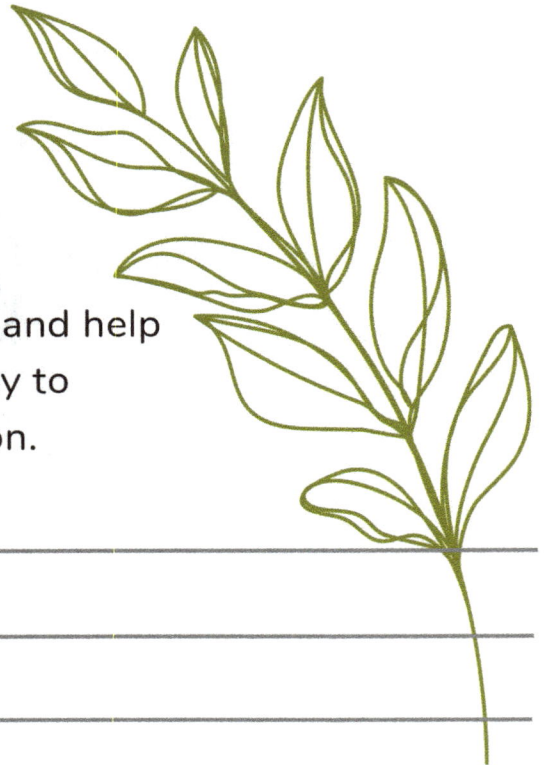

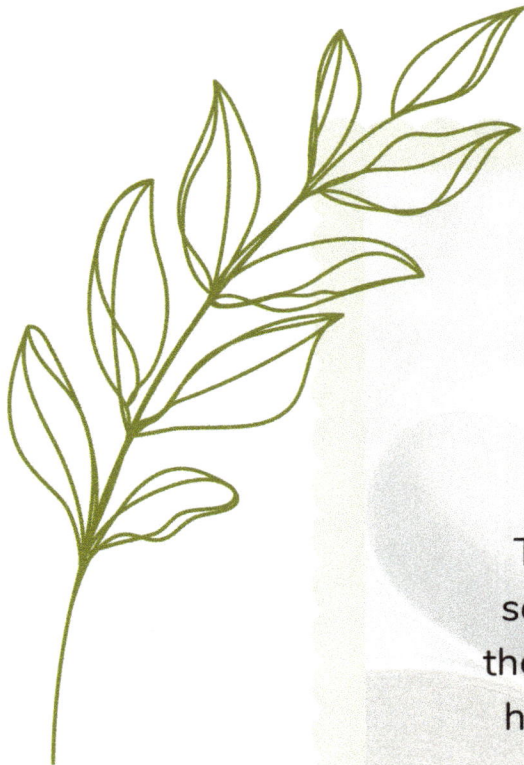

_____

_____

_____

Genesis 1:29

Then God said, 'I give you every seed-bearing plant on the face of the whole earth and every tree that has fruit with seed in it. They will be yours for food.

God's Word

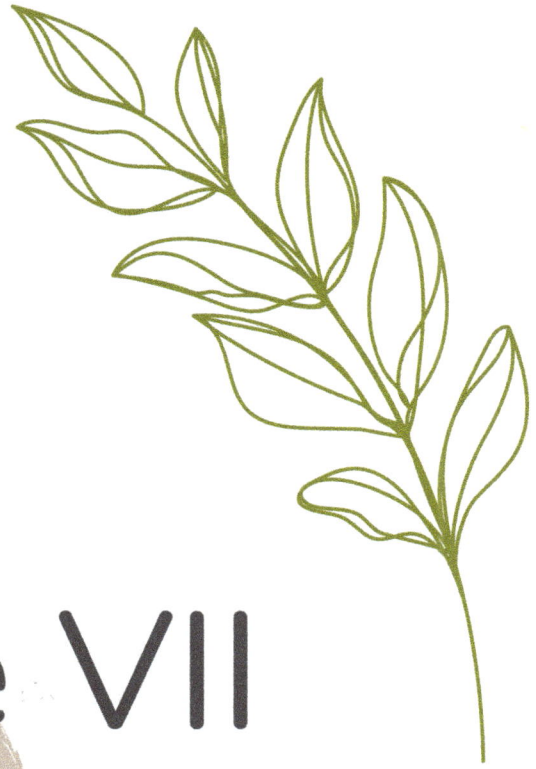

Phase VII

Balance
Blood Sugar

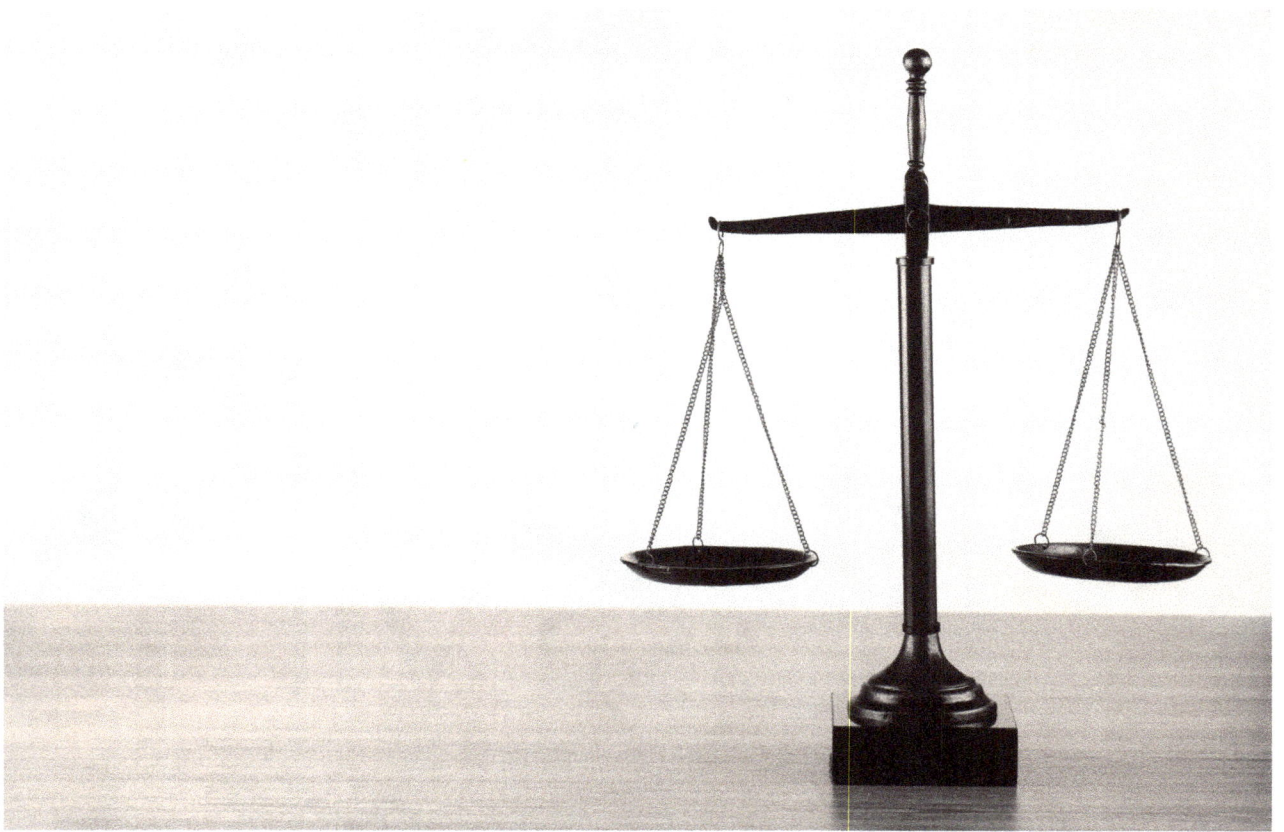

WHY IS IT IMPORTANT?

Balancing blood sugar is important for energy levels, mood stability, cognitive function, hunger and satiety, metabolic health, hormone balance, and digestive health.

But how do
we do this?

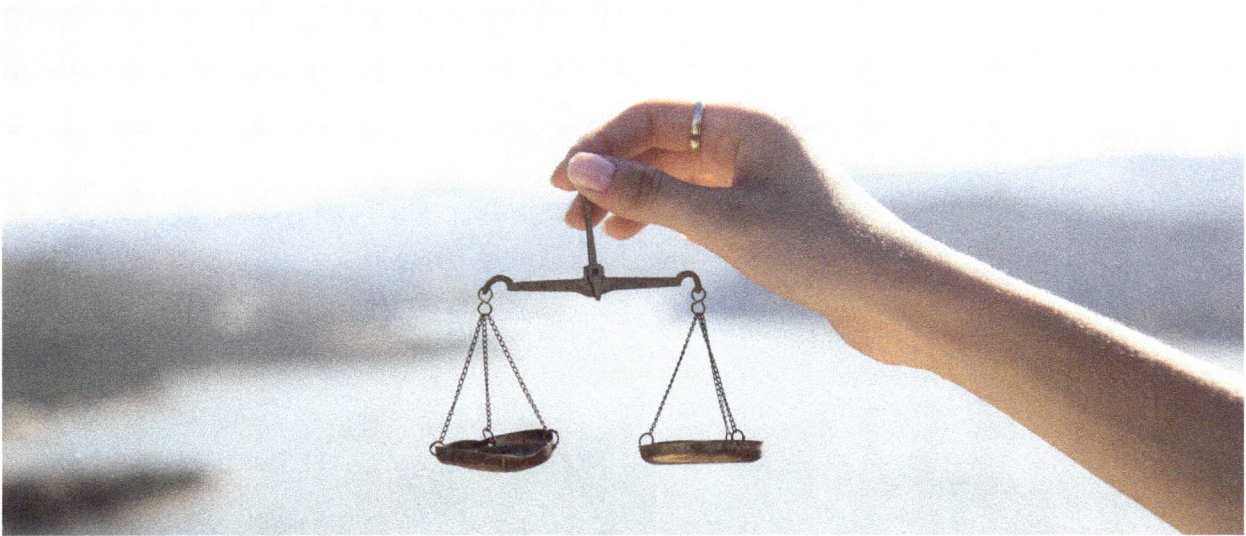

Action Steps

1

HEALTHY FATS

2

FIBER

3

Protein

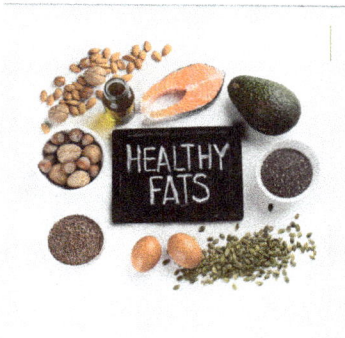

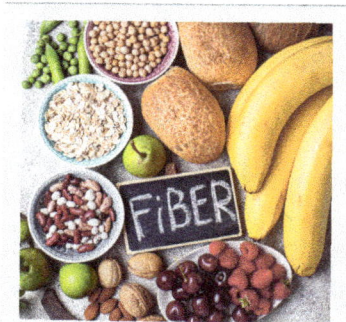

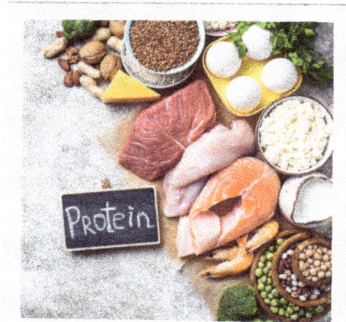

To balance your blood sugar, eat healthy fat, fiber, and protein for every meal including snacks.

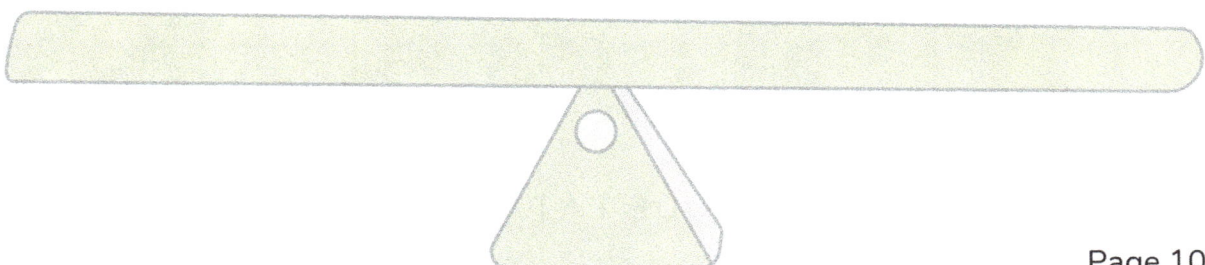

Currently

breakfast

Document what you ate:

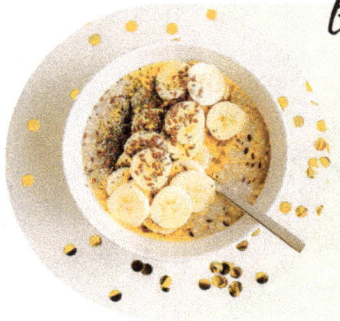

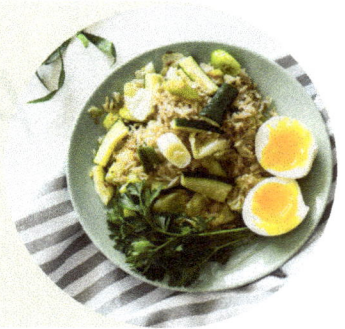

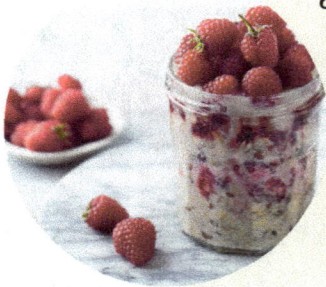

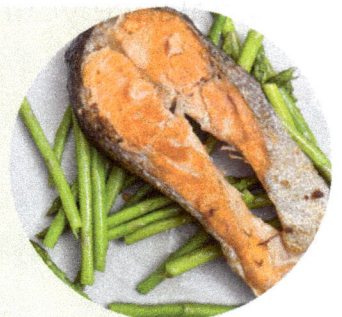

lunch

Document what you ate:

snack

Document what you ate:

dinner

Document what you ate:

DID EACH MEAL INCLUDE FAT, FIBER AND PROTEIN?

More Details...

THE POWER OF FAT, FIBER, AND PROTEIN

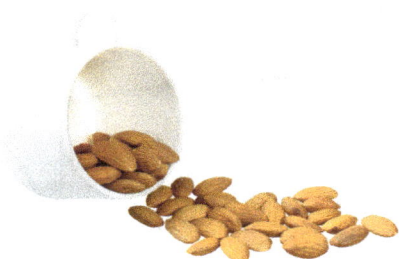

In order to balance blood sugar, provide satiety (feeling full after a meal), and balance energy throughout the day, try to aim for a mix of these factors at each meal and snack: Fat, Fiber, Protein.

> "
> Snacks and meals that contain a mix of fat, fiber and protein are more slowly digested than those containing only or mostly carbohydrates (including sugar). This slower digestion leads to a more even absorption of glucose (which all carbohydrates are broken down into), which in turn keeps your blood sugar levels balanced as well as helping you feel full longer. Feeling full longer will help eliminate those energy highs and lows (ie. crashes) that send you running for your next sugar fix.
>
> -Andrea Nakayama, Functional Nutrition Alliance
> "

Let's play a game and test your knowledge of Good Fats and Bad Fats.
Draw a line to connect the food item to either Good Fats or Bad Fats.

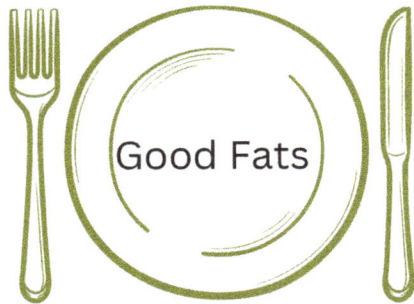

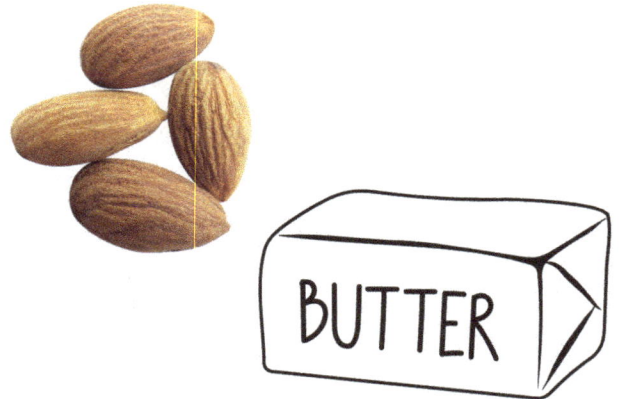

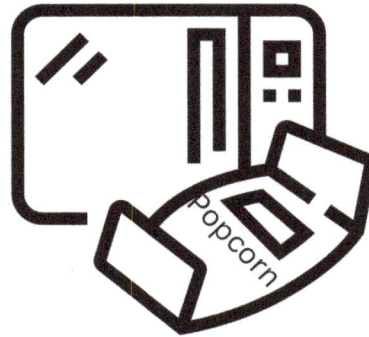

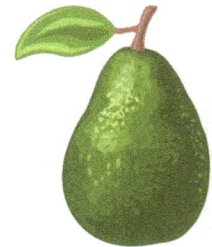

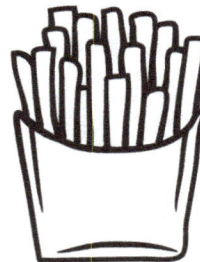

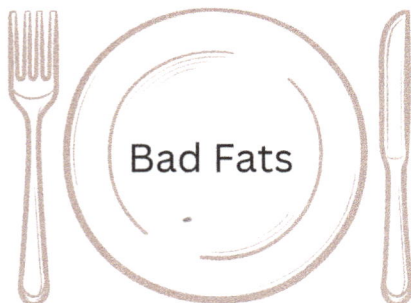

Good Fats

BUTTER

Popcorn

Bad Fats

Grass Fed Meats

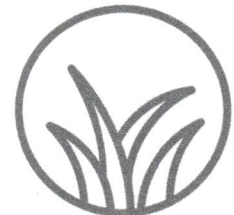

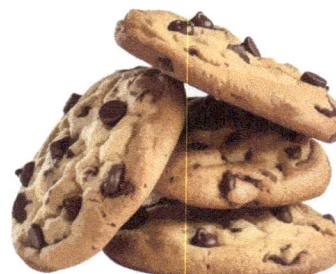

How did you do? Were there any surprises?
How about butter? Butter and ghee sources from organic or pasture-raised are a good fats, while margarine is a bad fat.

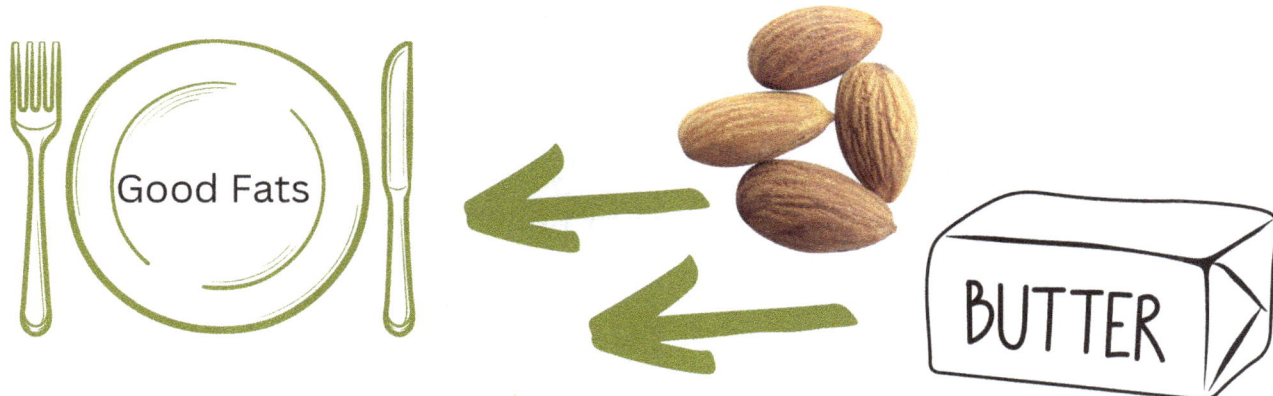

Good Fats

BUTTER

Microwave popcorn? Some microwave popcorns contain trans fats. Be sure to read the label. Better still, avoid using a microwave. Go back to the fun way of popping corn on the stove.

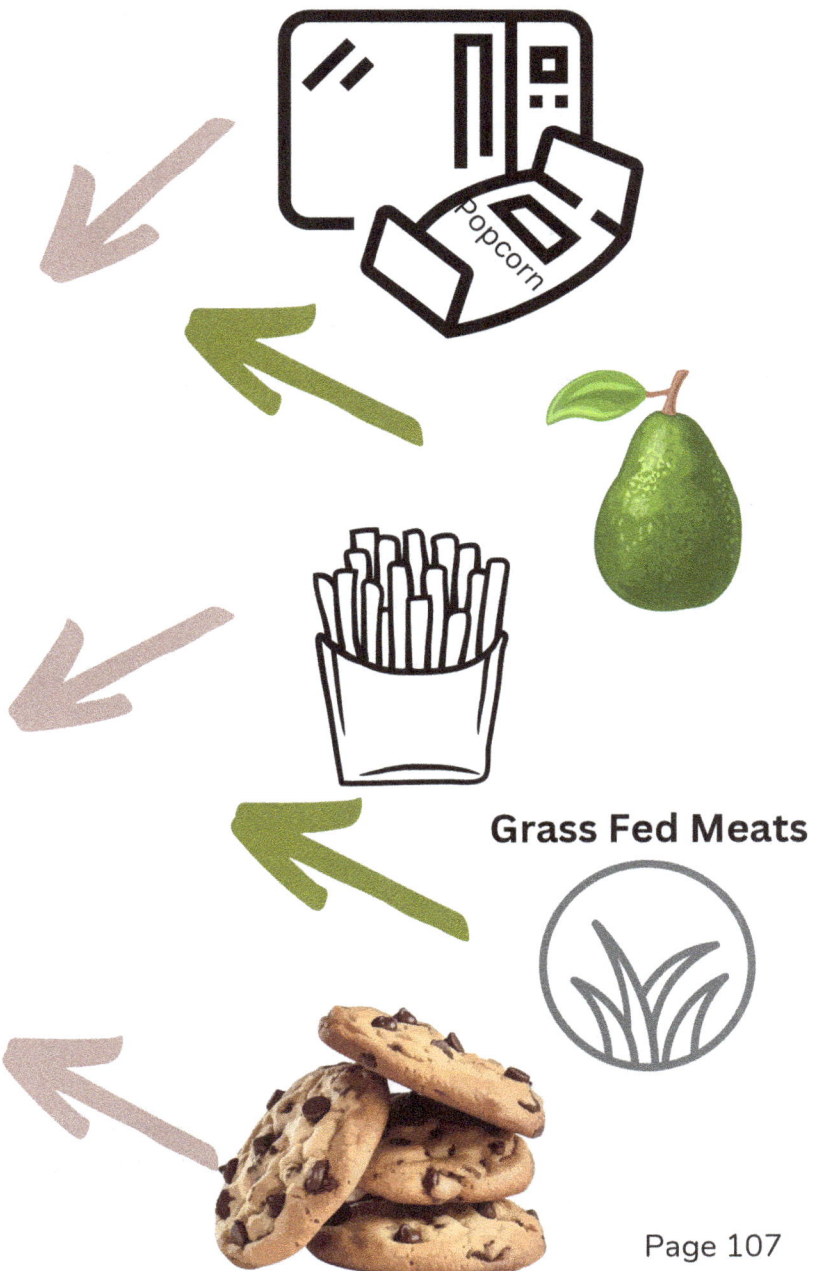

Popcorn

Grass Fed Meats

Bad Fats

Fats: The Good, The Bad, and The Ugly

Not all fats are bad. Our brain is made up of 60% fat. Our body needs good fats.

We encourage the intake of healthy fats from sources such as avocados, nuts, seeds, olive oil, and fatty fish, which provide essential fatty acids and support various bodily functions.

Fat plays important roles in our body such as:

1. Stores and carry nutrients around the body.
2. Provides physical insulation for organs.
3. Helps maintain body temperature.
4. Plays role in metabolism.
5. Leaves us feeling satisfied.
6. Helps maintain blood sugar (especially for those with diabetes).

> "
>
> The fats that heal, protect us from the fats that kill.
>
> -Andrea Nakayama, Functional Nutrition Alliance
>
> "

Our bodies need good fat, including:

Saturated Fat:

- Found mostly in animal fats and tropical oils such as coconut oil and palm oil.
  - Raw or organic butter (from grass-fed)
  - Raw or organic ghee (clarified butter where milk solids have been removed)
  - Lard from grass-fed
  - Coconut
- Solid at room temperature.
- Can be heated to higher temperatures without destroying their organic structure.
- Less likely to go rancid.
- Produces energy.
- Slows down absorption of your meals (so we can go longer without feeling hungry and helps maintain blood sugar).
- Helps maintain body heat and boost metabolism.
- The heart thrives on saturated fat in times of stress, but balance is important.

Monosaturated Fat:

- Found in:
  - olive oil (best at low-medium heat, not high heat)
  - olives
  - sesame oil
  - certain nuts
    - macadamia
    - pecans
    - Brazil nuts
    - almonds
    - cashews
    - pistachios
    - hazelnuts
  - certain legumes
    - peanuts
    - soybeans
  - avocados
  - canola oil (Dangerous for health! Yes to olive oil. No to canola oil.)
- Liquid at room temperature. Solid when refrigerated.
- Keeps arteries and skin healthy.
- Important heart protectors

Polyunsaturated Fat:

- Found mostly in
  - flax
  - hemp
  - chia
  - pumpkin
  - walnuts
  - fish
  - some meats
- Liquid at room temperature and in refrigerator.
- Required for normal cell, tissue, gland and organ function.
- Must be provided to the body from outside the body through food or supplements.

Our bodies do NOT need:

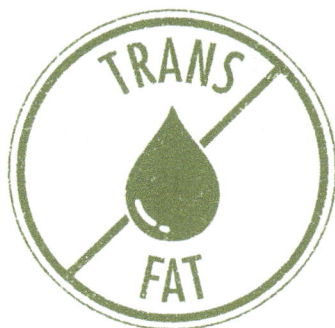

- **Partially Hydrogenated Oils:** These are the primary source of trans fats in processed foods. They are often found in:
  - Margarines and shortening
  - Baked goods (cookies, cakes, pastries)
  - Snack foods (crackers, microwave popcorn)
  - Fried foods (doughnuts, fried chicken)
- **Fast Food:** Many fast-food restaurants use partially hydrogenated oils for frying, which can contribute to trans fat content in their menu items.
- **Packaged Snacks:** Many commercially prepared snacks, like potato chips and certain types of candy, can contain trans fats.
- **Frozen Foods:** Some frozen meals and pizza may contain trans fats due to the use of partially hydrogenated oils.

It's important to read nutrition labels and ingredient lists carefully, as some products may contain trans fats even if they are labeled as "trans fat-free" (meaning they contain less than 0.5 grams per serving).

Fatty Acids

Omega-6

- Inflammatory
- Grains are higher in omega-6

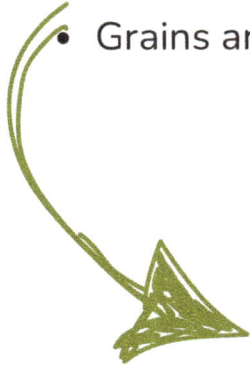

Omega-3

- Anti-inflammatory
- Found in fruits, vegetables, fatty fish, pastured eggs, free-range poultry, wild animals (elk, buffalo), walnuts, pumpkin seeds, hemp, flax, and chia seeds

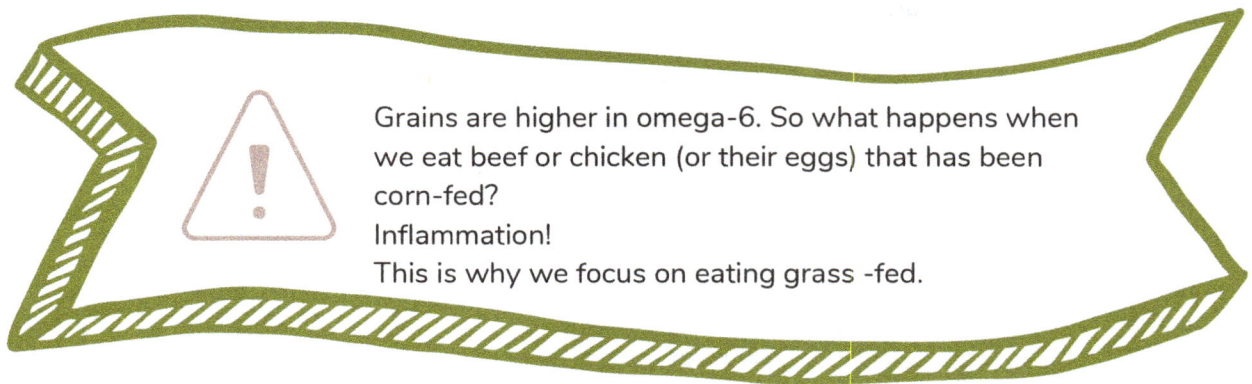

> ⚠️ Grains are higher in omega-6. So what happens when we eat beef or chicken (or their eggs) that has been corn-fed?
> Inflammation!
> This is why we focus on eating grass -fed.

Omega-6 : Omega-3

Omega-6 to Omega-3 ratio is important. The ideal ratio should be 1:1 or even 1:2.5 (Omega-6: Omega-3).

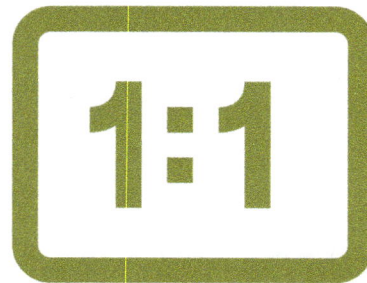

1:1

The American diet is 12:1 - 40:1! That's right. Some of us are eating foods higher in omega-6 causing our ratio to be as high as 40:1!

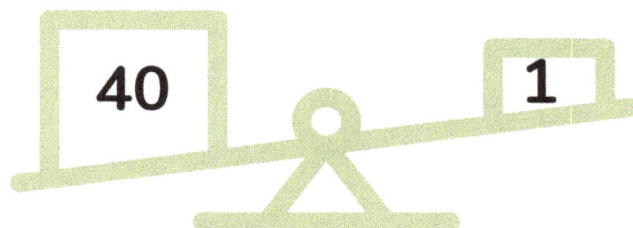

40   1

Fiber

Including fiber in your diet from whole grains, nuts and seeds, legumes, vegetables, and fruits (as opposed to an add-on in a processed food), is critical for the proper functioning of your gut.

Some important functions of fiber are:

- makes stool soft and bulky (easier to pass).

- speeds transit time through the colon.

- dilutes the effects of any toxic compounds in the intestine by moving them along and out of the system.

- helps to remove bad bacteria in the colon.

- feeds the good bacteria in the colon to allow for the production of vital nutrients such as B vitamins (essential for good brain health) and vitamin K (essential for bodily functions such as clotting)

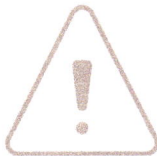

Always go slowly when making a dietary change, including one that increases fiber! Listen to your body and tune in to what works for you and your digestive system. If at first it doesn't feel great, then back down on the amount of fiber you are consuming and work your way up.

Protein

Protein comes from both animal and plant sources. Protein is critical to our ability to thrive and survive, allowing for maximal physiological repair and efficiency. The protein we consume provides amino acids our bodies need for a variety of critical functions. Protein is important because amino acids are a component in every cell and almost every fluid in our body and they provide the building blocks for bones, muscles, cartilage, blood, and skin.

Animal sources of protein include:
- beef
- chicken
- fish
- eggs
- bone broths

Plant sources include:
- nuts and nut butters
- seeds and seed butters
- soy (whole, fermented forms such as tempeh are preferred)
- legumes and lentils
- quinoa

Choose organic and grass-fed whenever possible.

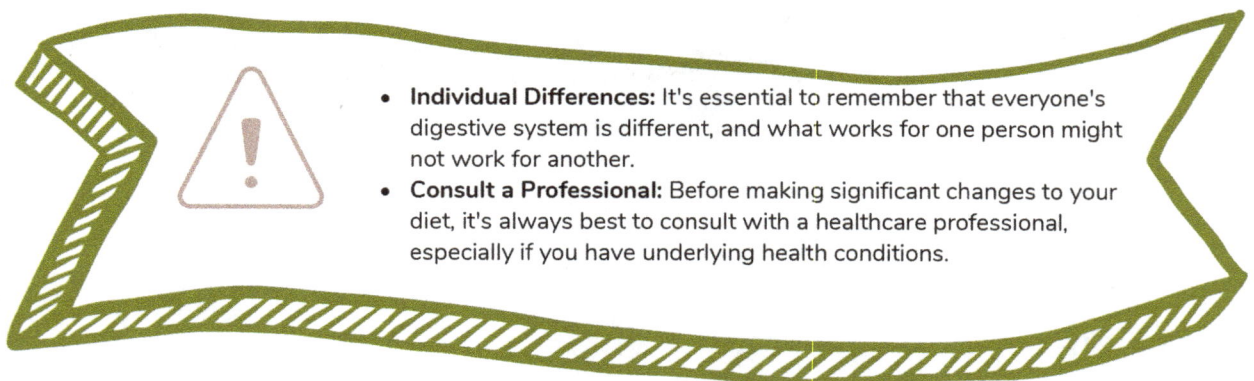

- **Individual Differences:** It's essential to remember that everyone's digestive system is different, and what works for one person might not work for another.
- **Consult a Professional:** Before making significant changes to your diet, it's always best to consult with a healthcare professional, especially if you have underlying health conditions.

New Way

WHAT CAN YOU ADD TO YOUR NORMAL MEALS TO INCLUDE FAT, FIBER AND PROTEIN?

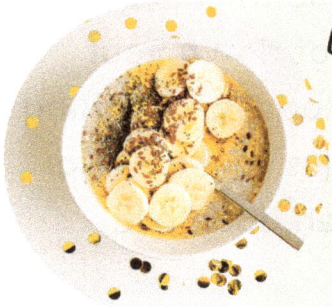

breakfast

lunch

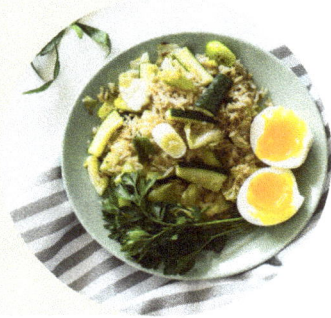

snack

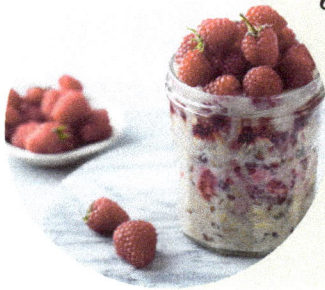

dinner

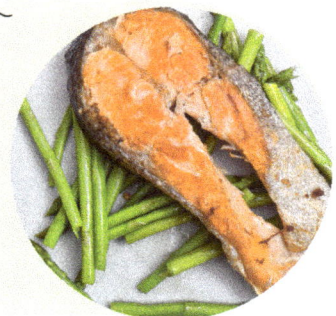

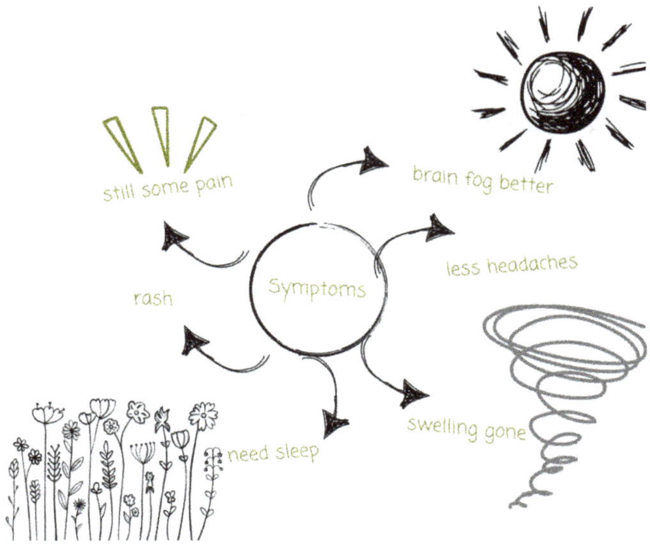

Track It!

Feel free to use the lines on this page to jot down your symptoms, mood, or anything else that comes to mind— or you could even doodle it!

still some pain

brain fog better

rash

Symptoms

less headaches

need sleep

swelling gone

Track It

Reflection Time

Honor God by taking care of your body. Take care of your body by eating balanced meals.

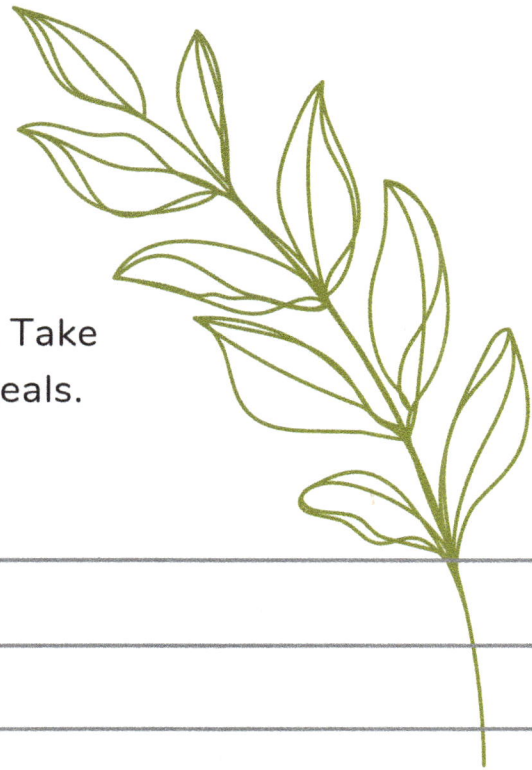

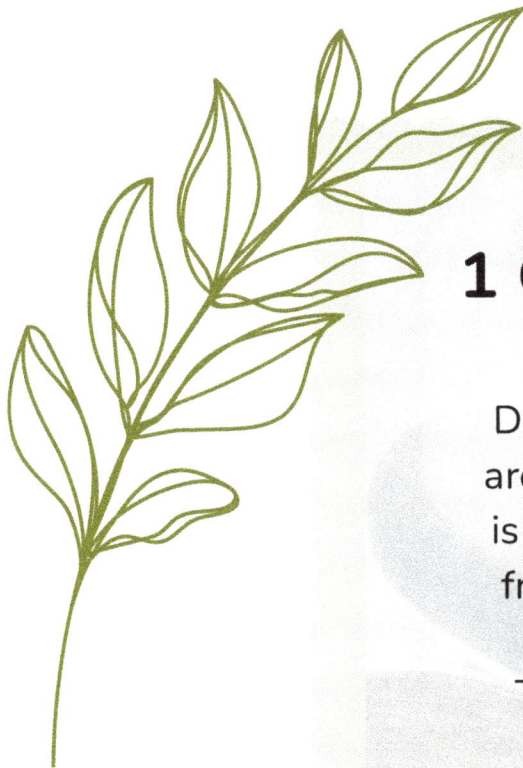

_____

_____

_____

1 Corinthians 6:19-20

Do you not know that your bodies are temples of the Holy Spirit, who is in you, whom you have received from God? You are not your own; you were bought at a price. Therefore, honor God with your bodies.

God's Word

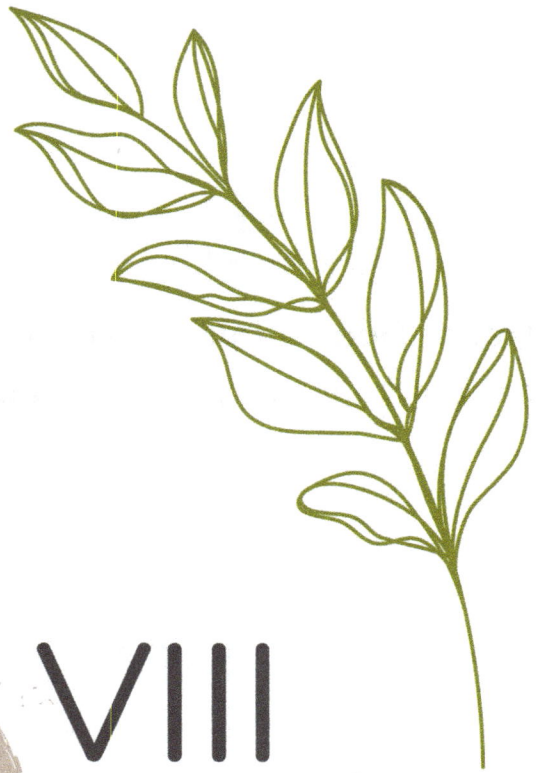

Phase VIII
Supplements

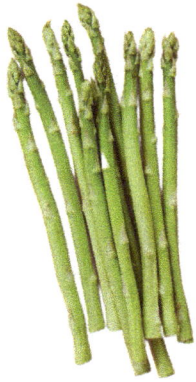

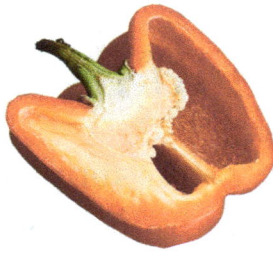

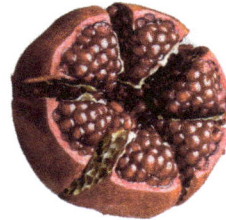

SUPPLEMENT PROTOCOL

Supplements are meant to "supplement" our diet. They can be helpful when we are unable to get needed nutrients or vitamins from our food, or when our body needs a boost due to deficiency.

The goal is to eat a healthy balanced diet to receive all of the nutrients we need.

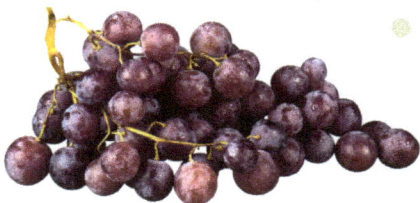

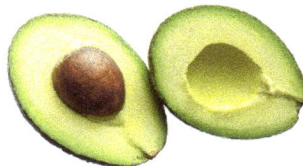

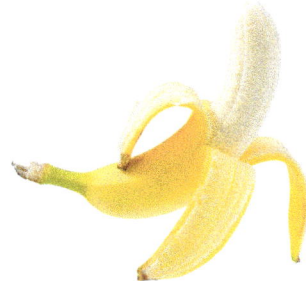

Think about it

What supplements are you
currently taking and why?

To Supplement...

More Details...

DISCOVER THE NUTRITIONAL TREASURES HIDDEN IN EVERYDAY FOODS

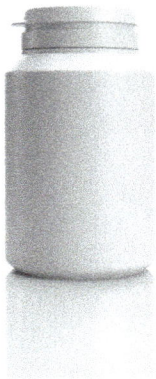

Before turning to supplements, take a look at the incredible variety of nutrients available in fruits, vegetables, whole grains, nuts, and more. From essential vitamins and minerals to antioxidants, fiber, healthy fats, and protein-rich foods, this guide highlights the natural goodness that supports your well-being.

ANTIOXIDANTS

Antioxidant-rich foods play a crucial role in protecting the body from oxidative stress and inflammation. Here is a list of foods that are known for their high antioxidant content:

- **Berries**
  - Blueberries
  - Strawberries
  - Raspberries
  - Blackberries
  - Cranberries
- **Nuts and seeds**
  - Walnuts
  - Almonds
  - Chia seeds
  - Flaxseeds
  - Sunflower seeds
- **Dark leafy greens**
  - Spinach
  - Kale
  - Swiss chard
  - Collard greens
- **Colorful vegetables**
  - Bell peppers (especially red, orange, and yellow)
  - Sweet potatoes
  - Carrots
  - Beets
- **Fruits**
  - Apples
  - Cherries
  - Grapes
  - Oranges
  - Kiwi
- **Herbs and spices**
  - Turmeric
  - Ginger
  - Cinnamon
  - Cloves
  - Oregano

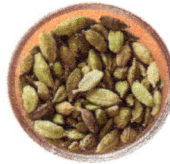

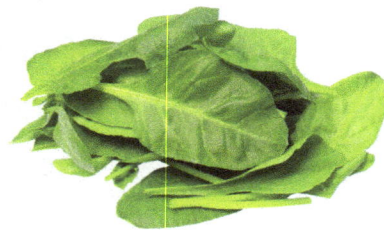

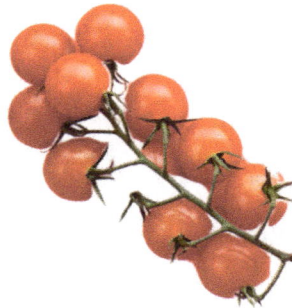

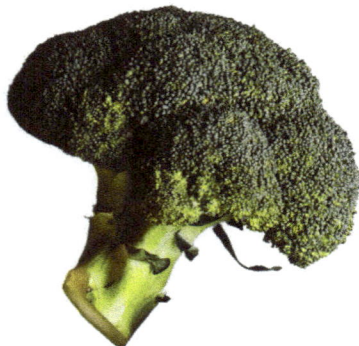

- **Whole grains**
  - Quinoa
  - Brown rice
  - Oats
- **Green tea**
  - Green tea is rich in catechins, powerful antioxidants.
- **Legumes**
  - Kidney beans
  - Black beans
  - Lentils
- **Fatty fish**
  - Salmon
  - Mackerel
  - Trout
- **Dark chocolate**
  - Choose dark chocolate with a high cocoa content for antioxidants.
- **Tomatoes**
  - Tomatoes contain lycopene, a potent antioxidant.

BETA CAROTENE

Beta-carotene is a precursor to vitamin A and is found in various fruits and vegetables.
Foods rich in beta-carotene:

- Carrots
- Sweet potatoes
- Butternut squash
- Pumpkin
- Spinach
- Kale
- Mangoes
- Cantaloupe
- Red and Yellow Bell Peppers
- Apricots
- Broccoli
- Papaya

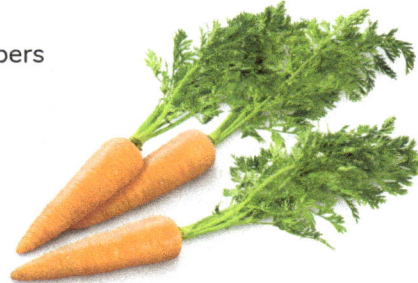

CURCUMIN

Curcumin is the active compound found in turmeric, a spice known for its anti-inflammatory and antioxidant properties.
Foods and dishes that commonly include turmeric, thus providing curcumin:

- Curry powder
- Turmeric tea
- Golden milk
- Indian cuisine
- Turmeric rice
- Add turmeric to smoothies, roasted vegetables, soup, hummus

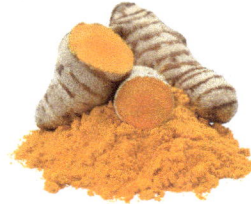

DIGESTIVE ENZYMES

Digestive enzymes are produced naturally by the body. However, some people may have deficiencies in certain digestive enzymes or conditions that impair enzyme production, leading to digestive issues. Foods that will aid in digestion include:

- Pineapple
- Papaya
- Kiwi
- Mango
- Honey
- Avocado
- Sauerkraut
- Kefir
- Yogurt
- Miso

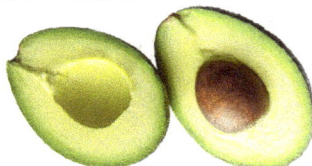

FATTY ACIDS

Incorporating healthy fatty acids into your diet is crucial for overall well-being. Here's a list of foods rich in healthy fatty acids, including omega-3 and omega-6 fatty acids:

Foods High in Omega-3 Fatty Acids:

1. Fatty Fish: Salmon, mackerel, trout, sardines, and herring are excellent sources.
2. Flaxseeds: Ground flaxseeds or flaxseed oil provide a plant-based source of omega-3s.
3. Chia Seeds: These tiny seeds are rich in alpha-linolenic acid (ALA), a type of omega-3 fatty acid.
4. Walnuts: Walnuts are a convenient and tasty nut high in omega-3s.
5. Hemp Seeds: Hemp seeds contain a good balance of omega-3 and omega-6 fatty acids.

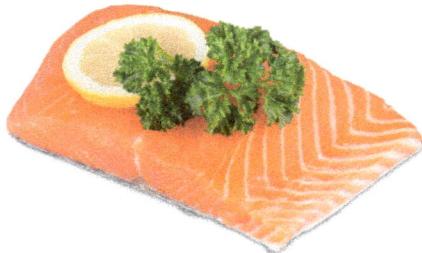

Foods High in Omega-6 Fatty Acids:

1. Sunflower Seeds: These seeds are a great source of omega-6 fatty acids.
2. Safflower Oil: Cooking with safflower oil can contribute to omega-6 intake.
3. Pumpkin Seeds: Pumpkin seeds, or pepitas, provide a mix of omega-6 and omega-3 fatty acids.
4. Nuts and Seeds: Almonds, pine nuts, and sesame seeds are examples of nuts and seeds high in omega-6s.

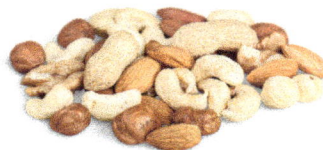

Other Healthy Fats:

1. Avocado: Avocados are rich in monounsaturated fats, which are heart-healthy.
2. Olive Oil: Extra virgin olive oil is a source of monounsaturated fats and has numerous health benefits.
3. Coconut Oil: While high in saturated fat, coconut oil contains medium-chain triglycerides (MCTs) with potential health benefits.
4. Dark Chocolate: Dark chocolate with high cocoa content contains healthy fats, especially monounsaturated fats.
5. Eggs: Eggs, especially the yolk, contain various healthy fats and nutrients.

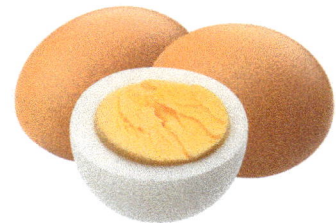

FIBER

Fiber is essential for healthy digestion, as it helps keep the digestive tract moving, prevents constipation, and supports gut health. It also aids in blood sugar control, lowers cholesterol, and can promote a feeling of fullness, supporting weight management and overall well-being.

- **Whole grains**
  - Oats
  - Quinoa
  - Brown rice
  - Barley
  - Bulgur
  - Whole wheat
- **Legumes**
  - Lentils
  - Chickpeas
  - Black beans
  - Kidney beans
- **Vegetables**
  - Broccoli
  - Carrots
  - Brussels sprouts
  - Spinach
  - Sweet potatoes
  - Kale
- **Fruits**
  - Apples
  - Pears
  - Berries (raspberries, blackberries, strawberries)
  - Bananas
  - Oranges
- **Nuts and Seeds**
  - Almonds
  - Chia seeds
  - Flaxseeds
  - Sunflower seeds
  - Walnuts

- **Whole grain bread and pasta**
  - Whole wheat bread
  - Whole grain pasta
- **Dried Fruits**
  - Raisins
  - Prunes
  - Apricots
- **Root vegetables**
  - Potatoes (with skin)
  - Beets
  - Turnips
  - Radishes
- **Popcorn**
  - Air-popped popcorn

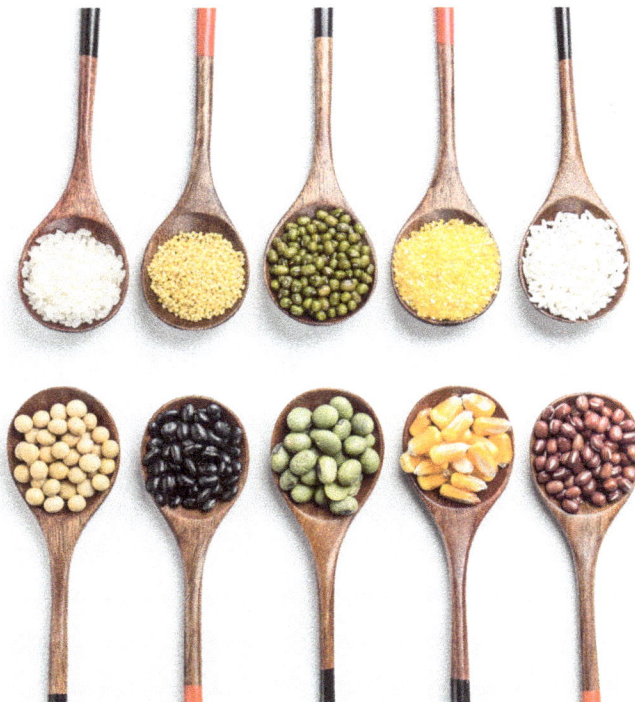

IRON

Iron is an essential mineral that plays a crucial role in various bodily functions, including transporting oxygen in the blood. Foods that are good sources of iron:

- **Red meat (grass fed when possible)**
  - Beef
  - Lamb
  - Pork
- **Poultry (pastured raised when possible)**
  - Chicken
  - Turkey
- **Fish (wild caught)**
  - Salmon
  - Tuna
  - Sardines
- **Shellfish**
  - Oysters
  - Clams
  - Mussels
  - Shrimp
- **Legumes**
  - Lentils
  - Chickpeas (garbanzo beans)
  - Black beans
  - Kidney beans
- **Nuts and Seeds**
  - Pumpkin seeds
  - Sesame seeds
  - Cashews

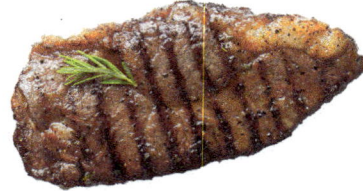

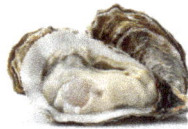

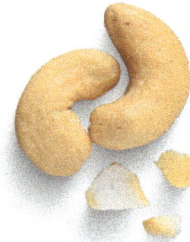

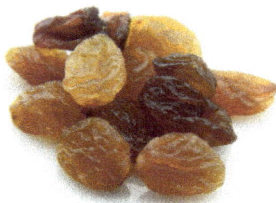

- **Quinoa**
  - Quinoa is a seed that is often considered a whole grain and contains iron.
- **Dark leafy greens**
  - Spinach
  - Kale
  - Swiss chard
  - Collard greens
- **Dried fruits**
  - Apricots
  - Raisins
  - Prunes
- **Organ Meats (in Moderation):**
  - Liver (beef, chicken, lamb) is a rich source of iron, but it should be consumed in moderation due to its high vitamin A content.

L-GLUTAMINE

L-glutamine is an amino acid that plays a crucial role in various bodily functions, including supporting the immune system and maintaining the health of the digestive tract. Foods that contain L-glutamine:

- **Animal Proteins (grass-fed, pasture raised, wild caught):**
  - Beef
  - Chicken
  - Fish
  - Turkey
  - Eggs
- **Dairy Products:**
  - Milk
  - Yogurt
  - Cheese
- **Plant-Based Proteins:**
  - Beans (especially soybeans)
  - Lentils
  - Peas
- **Nuts and Seeds:**
  - Almonds
  - Walnuts
  - Sunflower seeds
- **Whole Grains:**
  - Quinoa
  - Brown rice
  - Oats
- **Vegetables:**
  - Cabbage
  - Spinach
  - Parsley
- **Fruits:**
  - Avocado
  - Papaya
- **Fermented Foods:**
  - Yogurt (contains probiotics that support gut health)
  - Kimchi
  - Miso

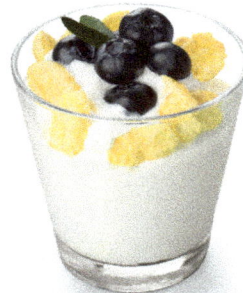

MAGNESIUM

Magnesium is an essential mineral that plays a vital role in various physiological functions in the body. Here are some foods that are good sources of magnesium:

- **Leafy Green Vegetables:**
  - Spinach
  - Kale
  - Swiss chard
  - Collard greens
- **Nuts and Seeds:**
  - Almonds
  - Cashews
  - Pumpkin seeds
  - Sunflower seeds
- **Whole Grains:**
  - Brown rice
  - Quinoa
  - Oats
  - Whole wheat
- **Legumes:**
  - Black beans
  - Chickpeas
  - Lentils
- **Fish (wild caught):**
  - Salmon
  - Mackerel
  - Halibut
- **Dairy Products:**
  - Yogurt
  - Milk
  - Cheese
- **Dark Chocolate**
- **Tofu**
- **Figs**
- **Potatoes**
- **Seaweed**
- **Whole Grain Bread**
- **Edamame**
- **Bananas**
- **Avocado**

PROTEIN

- **Meat (grass-fed):**
  - Beef
  - Pork
  - Lamb
  - Venison
- **Poultry (pasture raised):**
  - Chicken
  - Turkey
  - Duck
- **Fish (wild caught):**
  - Salmon
  - Tuna
  - Trout
  - Cod
  - Haddock
- **Seafood:**
  - Shrimp
  - Crab
  - Lobster
  - Mussels
  - Clams
- **Eggs:**
  - Eggs are a complete protein source.
- **Dairy:**
  - Milk
  - Yogurt
  - Cheese
  - Cottage cheese
  - Greek yogurt
- **Plant-Based Proteins:**
  - Tofu
  - Tempeh
  - Edamame
  - Lentils
  - Chickpeas
- **Legumes:**
  - Black beans
  - Kidney beans
  - Pinto beans
  - Navy beans

- **Nuts:**
  - Almonds
  - Walnuts
  - Pistachios
  - Cashews
- **Seeds:**
  - Chia seeds
  - Flaxseeds
  - Sunflower seeds
  - Pumpkin seeds
- **Grains:**
  - Quinoa
  - Brown rice
  - Barley
  - Bulgur
  - Oats
- **Dairy Alternatives:**
  - Plant-based milk (soy, almond, oat, etc.)
  - Plant-based yogurt
  - Plant-based cheese
- **Protein Supplements:**
  - Whey protein
  - Casein protein
  - Pea protein
  - Hemp protein
  - Rice protein

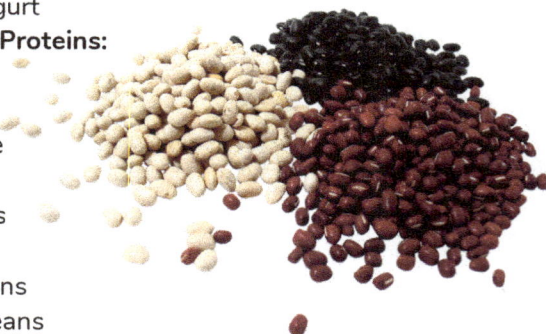

SELENIUM

Selenium is an essential mineral that plays a crucial role in various bodily functions, including antioxidant defense and supporting the immune system. Here is a list of foods that are good sources of selenium:

- **Brazil Nuts:**
  - Eating just a few nuts can provide your daily recommended intake.
- **Fish:**
  - Tuna
  - Halibut
  - Sardines
  - Salmon
- **Shellfish:**
  - Shrimp
  - Crab
  - Lobster
- **Meat:**
  - Beef
  - Pork
  - Lamb
- **Poultry:**
  - Chicken
  - Turkey
- **Eggs:**
  - Eggs, especially the yolks
- **Whole Grains:**
  - Brown rice
  - Whole wheat bread
  - Oats
- **Dairy:**
  - Milk
  - Yogurt
- **Seeds:**
  - Sunflower seeds
- **Legumes:**
  - Lentils
  - Chickpeas
  - Black beans
- **Vegetables:**
  - Spinach and other leafy greens
  - Mushrooms: Some varieties of mushrooms, such as shiitake and white button mushrooms

TYROSINE

Tyrosine is an amino acid that is a precursor to several important neurotransmitters, including dopamine, norepinephrine, and adrenaline. Including foods rich in tyrosine in your diet can support the production of these neurotransmitters. At the top of the list of foods high in tyrosine is spirulina! Spirulina is a type of blue-green algae. Here are some other foods that are good sources of tyrosine:

- **Meat:**
  - Chicken
  - Turkey
  - Beef
  - Pork
  - Buffalo
  - Elk
  - Quail
  - Duck
- **Fish:**
  - Salmon
  - Tuna
- **Dairy:**
  - Cheese
  - Yogurt
  - Milk
- **Eggs:**
  - Particularly egg whites
- **Soy Products:**
  - Tofu
  - Tempeh
  - Though we can't advocate the consumption of many soy products, especially when we're talking about hormone issues, soy does contain some good amounts of tyrosine.
- **Nuts and Seeds:**
  - Almonds
  - Peanuts
  - Pumpkin seeds
  - Sesame seeds

- **Beans and Legumes:**
  - Lentils
  - Chickpeas
- **Whole Grains:**
  - Oats
  - Wheat
  - Quinoa
- **Fruits and Vegetables:**
  - Bananas
  - Avocados
  - Spinach
  - Mustard greens

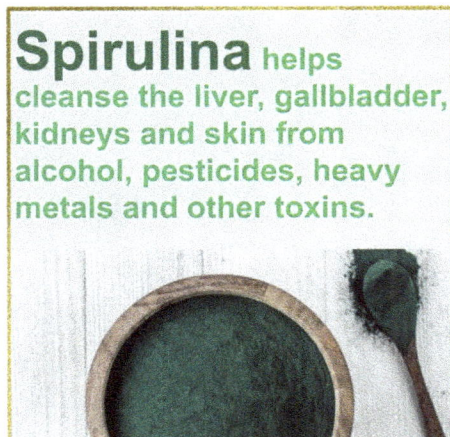

Spirulina helps cleanse the liver, gallbladder, kidneys and skin from alcohol, pesticides, heavy metals and other toxins.

VITAMINS

Vitamin A	Vitamin B
• Carrots • Sweet Potatoes • Spinach • Kale • Broccoli • Butternut Squash • Cantaloupe • Red Bell Peppers • Mango • Apricots • Eggs • Liver (Note: Liver is very high in vitamin A, so consume it in moderation)	• **B1 (Thiamine):** Supports energy metabolism and nerve function. Found in whole grains, nuts, seeds, and legumes. • **B2 (Riboflavin):** Important for energy production and maintaining healthy skin. Found in dairy products, lean meats, and green leafy vegetables. • **B3 (Niacin):** Supports energy production, skin health, and nervous system function. Found in meat, fish, poultry, whole grains, and legumes. • **B5 (Pantothenic Acid):** Essential for the synthesis of fatty acids and energy production. Found in a wide variety of foods, including meat, whole grains, and vegetables. • **B6 (Pyridoxine):** Involved in amino acid metabolism, neurotransmitter synthesis, and red blood cell formation. Found in meat, fish, poultry, bananas, and potatoes. • **B7 (Biotin):** Important for metabolism, particularly of carbohydrates and fats. Found in eggs, nuts, seeds, and some vegetables. • **B9 (Folate/Folic Acid):** Crucial for DNA synthesis and cell division. Found in leafy greens, legumes, citrus fruits, and fortified grains. • **B12 (Cobalamin):** Vital for red blood cell formation, neurological function, and DNA synthesis. Found in animal products such as meat, fish, eggs, and dairy.

Vitamin C

- **Citrus Fruits:**
  - Oranges
  - Grapefruits
  - Lemons
  - Limes
  - Tangerines
- **Berries:**
  - Strawberries
  - Blueberries
  - Raspberries
  - Blackberries
  - Cranberries
- **Tropical Fruits:**
  - Pineapple
  - Mango
  - Papaya
  - Guava
  - Kiwi
- **Melons:**
  - Watermelon
  - Cantaloupe
  - Honeydew

- **Other Fruits:**
  - Apples
  - Pears
  - Peaches
  - Plums
- **Vegetables:**
  - Red and Green Bell Peppers
  - Broccoli
  - Brussels Sprouts
  - Spinach
  - Kale
  - Tomatoes
- **Cruciferous Vegetables:**
  - Cauliflower
  - Cabbage
  - Bok Choy
- **Other Vegetables:**
  - Potatoes
  - Sweet Potatoes
  - Carrots
- **Herbs:**
  - Parsley
  - Cilantro
  - Thyme

VITAMINS CONT.

Vitamin D	Vitamin E
<ul><li>**Fatty Fish:**<ul><li>Salmon</li><li>Mackerel</li><li>Sardines</li><li>Herring</li><li>Trout</li></ul></li><li>**Cod Liver Oil:**<ul><li>Cod liver oil is a highly concentrated source of vitamin D.</li></ul></li><li>**Egg Yolks:**<ul><li>Eggs contain small amounts of vitamin D, with higher concentrations in the yolks.</li></ul></li><li>**Cheese:**<ul><li>Some types of cheese, such as Swiss and cheddar, contain small amounts of vitamin D.</li></ul></li><li>**Beef Liver:**<ul><li>Beef liver is a good source of various nutrients, including vitamin D.</li></ul></li><li>**Mushrooms:**<ul><li>Mushrooms naturally contain small amounts of vitamin D.</li></ul></li></ul>	<ul><li>**Nuts and Seeds**<ul><li>Almonds: One of the best sources of vitamin E. A handful (about 1 ounce) of almonds provides a significant portion of your daily needs.</li><li>Sunflower Seeds: High in vitamin E, with a quarter-cup providing a substantial amount.</li><li>Hazelnuts: Another excellent source of vitamin E.</li><li>Pine Nuts: A good source of vitamin E, often used in salads and pesto.</li></ul></li><li>**Oils**<ul><li>Wheat germ oil: One of the richest sources of vitamin E.</li><li>Olive oil: While not as high as sunflower or wheat germ oil, it still provides a decent amount of vitamin E.</li></ul></li><li>**Vegetables**<ul><li>Spinach: Dark leafy greens like spinach are good sources of vitamin E.</li><li>Swiss chard: Another leafy green high in vitamin E.</li><li>Broccoli: Contains a modest amount of vitamin E.</li><li>Avocado: A great source of healthy fats and vitamin E.</li></ul></li><li>**Fruits**<ul><li>Kiwi: Contains vitamin E along with other essential nutrients.</li><li>Mango: A tropical fruit rich in vitamin E.</li><li>Tomatoes: While not extremely high in vitamin E, they contribute to overall intake when included in the diet.</li></ul></li><li>**Grains and Other Sources**<ul><li>Whole grains: Foods like whole wheat and oats contain vitamin E</li><li>Eggs: Provide some vitamin E along with other essential nutrients.</li><li>Shellfish: Certain types of shellfish, though not applicable in your case due to allergies, are also good sources.</li></ul></li></ul>

Vitamin K

- **Leafy Green Vegetables:**
  - Kale
  - Spinach
  - Swiss chard
  - Collard greens
  - Turnip greens
  - Broccoli
- **Cruciferous Vegetables:**
  - Brussels sprouts
  - Cabbage
  - Cauliflower
- **Herbs:**
  - Parsley
  - Cilantro
  - Basil
- **Green Lettuce:**
  - Romaine lettuce
  - Iceberg lettuce
  - Leaf lettuce
- **Vegetables:**
  - Asparagus
  - Okra
  - Green beans
  - Peas
- **Fruits:**
  - Kiwi
  - Blueberries
  - Grapes
- **Meat:**
  - Pork
  - Beef liver
- **Dairy:**
  - Cheese, especially hard cheeses like cheddar and Swiss
- **Oils:**
  - Olive oil
- **Fish:**
  - Salmon
- **Natto:**
  - Fermented soybean product
- **Nuts:**
  - Cashews
  - Pistachios

ZINC

- **Meat (grass-fed):**
  - Beef
  - Pork
  - Lamb
- **Poultry (pasture raised):**
  - Chicken
  - Turkey
- **Seafood:**
  - Oysters (highly rich in zinc)
  - Crab
  - Lobster
  - Shrimp
  - Fish (wild caught)
- **Dairy:**
  - Milk
  - Cheese
  - Yogurt
- **Eggs:**
  - Eggs are a moderate source of zinc.
- **Legumes:**
  - Lentils
  - Chickpeas
  - Black beans
- **Nuts and Seeds:**
  - Pumpkin seeds (pepitas)
  - Cashews
  - Almonds
  - Sesame seeds and butter
  - Peanuts
- **Whole Grains:**
  - Quinoa
  - Brown rice
  - Oats
- **Vegetables:**
  - Spinach
  - Kale
  - Mushrooms
- **Pumpkin and Squash Seeds:**
  - These seeds, often consumed as snacks, are rich in zinc.
- **Dark Chocolate:**
  - Dark chocolate contains some zinc.

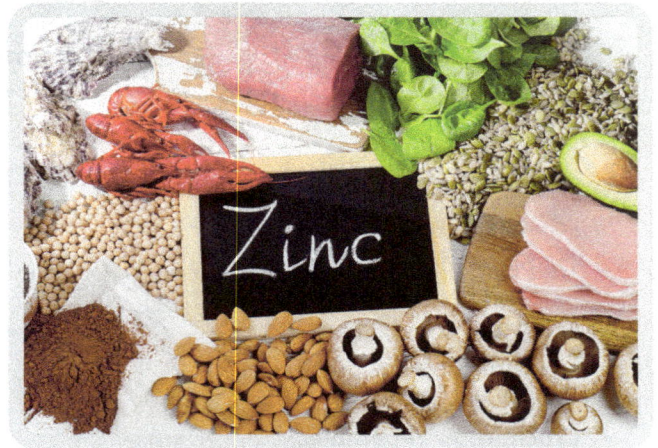

PROBIOTICS, PREBIOTICS, AND ENZYMES

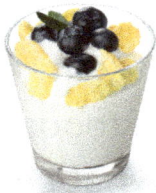

What are probiotics, prebiotics, and enzymes?
Why do I need them?
How do I get them?

Let's talk about enzymes, little helpers in our body that break down food into tiny pieces that we can use. It's like having tiny workers in our digestive system! These workers chop up our food into smaller bits so our body can easily soak up the good stuff, like nutrients. Enzymes are like the superheroes that make our food ready for our bodies to use!

Enzymes are naturally present in our bodies, produced by various organs like the salivary glands, stomach, and pancreas. Additionally, raw and fermented foods, such as fruits, vegetables, and yogurt, contain enzymes that can support digestion. While our bodies produce enzymes, incorporating enzyme-rich foods into our diet may provide additional support for the digestive process.

PROBIOTICS

Definition:
- Probiotics are beneficial bacteria that promote a healthy balance of microorganisms in the gut.
- They can be found in fermented foods like yogurt, kefir, sauerkraut, and kimchi.

Function:
- Help maintain a healthy balance of gut bacteria
- Support the immune system
- Aid in digestion and nutrient absorption
- May help alleviate symptoms of certain digestive disorders like irritable bowel syndrome (IBS) and inflammatory disease (IBD)

Sources:
- Fermented foods such as yogurt, kefir, sauerkraut, kimchi, and miso
- Probiotic supplements

PREBIOTICS

Definition:
- Prebiotics are non-digestible fibers and compounds that feed the beneficial bacteria (probiotics) in your gut, promoting their growth and activity.

Function:
- Serve as food for probiotics, helping them thrive and maintain a healthy gut microbiome
- Improve digestion and absorption of nutrients
- May help regulate bowel movements and support overall gut health

Sources:
- High-fiber foods such as garlic, onions, leeks, asparagus, bananas, and whole grains
- Prebiotic supplements

ENZYMES

Definition:
- Digestive enzymes are proteins produced by the body that help break down food into smaller, absorbable nutrients.

Function:
- Facilitate the breakdown of carbohydrates, proteins, and fats into their respective monomers (sugars, amino acids, and fatty acids)
- Improve the efficiency of nutrient absorption
- Reduce symptoms of indigestion, such as bloating, gas, and discomfort

Sources:
- The body naturally produces digestive enzymes in the salivary glands, stomach, pancreas, and small intestine.
- Enzyme-rich foods such as pineapples (bromelain), papayas (papain), and fermented foods
- Digestive enzyme supplements

Think about it

Are there supplements that you may not need? Are you able to obtain sufficient nutrients and vitamins with whole foods instead? Jot down what changes you can make in your diet to obtain needed nutrients and vitamins.

Make changes that you feel are right for you, then track it.

Or Not to Supplement

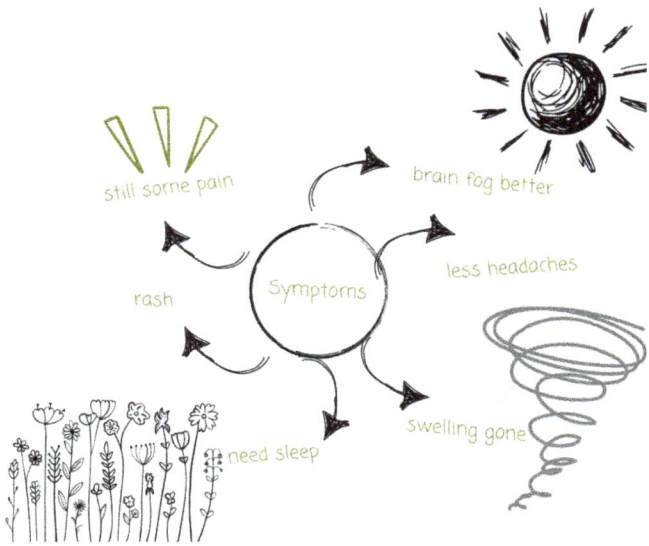

Track It!

Feel free to use the lines on this page to jot down your symptoms, mood, or anything else that comes to mind— or you could even doodle it!

still some pain

brain fog better

rash

Symptoms

less headaches

need sleep

swelling gone

Track It

Reflection Time

Supplements are necessary for a lot of people. Just make sure that what you are taking is necessary for you.

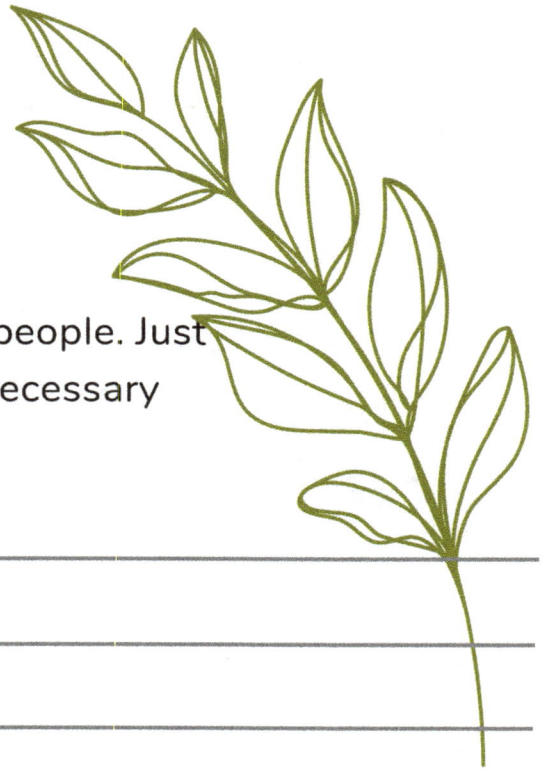

_____

_____

_____

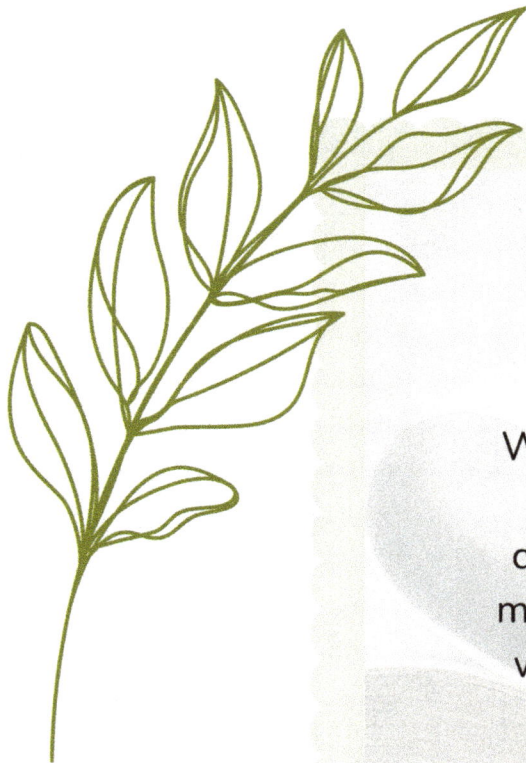

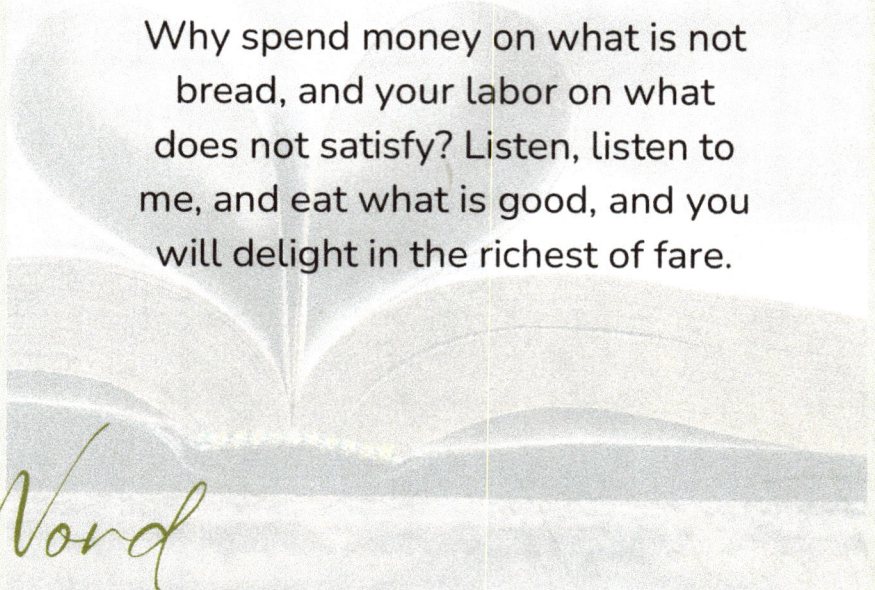

Isaiah 55:2

Why spend money on what is not bread, and your labor on what does not satisfy? Listen, listen to me, and eat what is good, and you will delight in the richest of fare.

God's Word

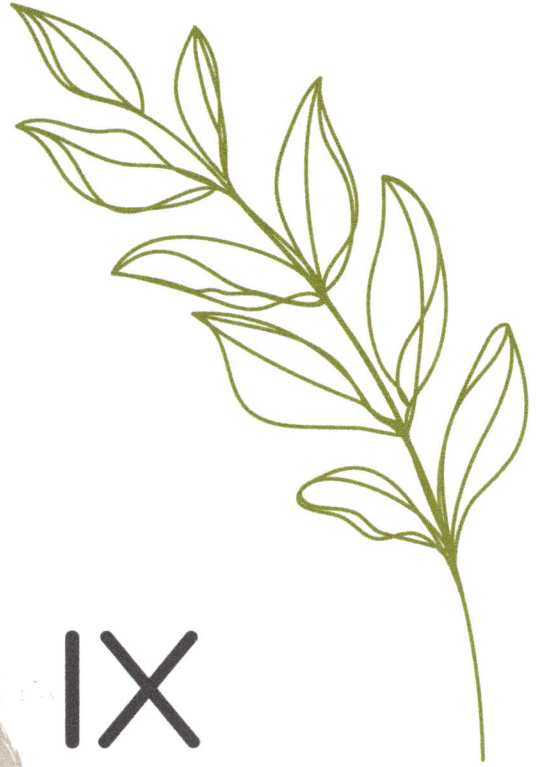

Phase IX
Cravings

What do you crave?

Jot down the things that you crave, and if you notice anything that triggers the craving.

I crave chocolate after eating a healthy salad.

Cravings

Your Body is Talking to You

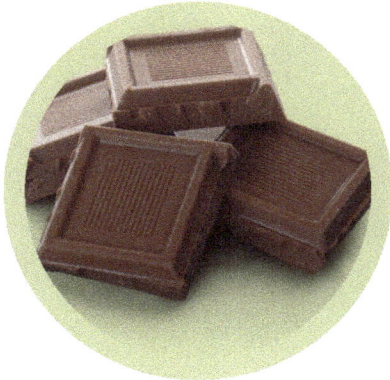

1 Chocolate

Chocolate, especially dark chocolate, is rich in magnesium, and craving it may be an indicator of a deficiency in this mineral.

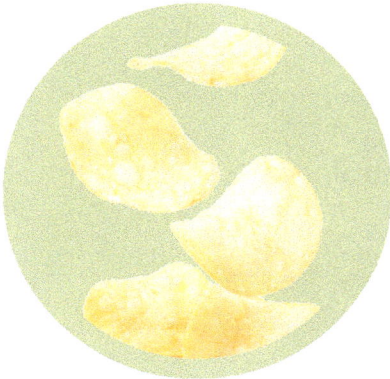

2 Salty Foods

Craving salty foods can be an indicator that the body needs potassium, sodium, or other electrolytes.

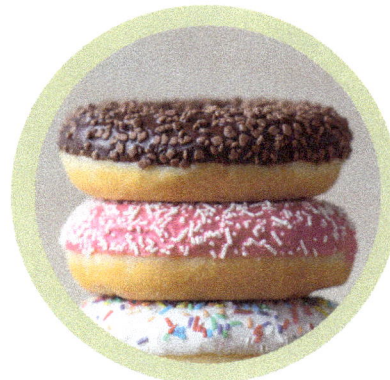

3 Sugary Foods

Craving sweets may indicate that your blood sugar has dropped, and your body needs a quick source of energy. Remember to include fat, fiber, and protein when selecting a snack.

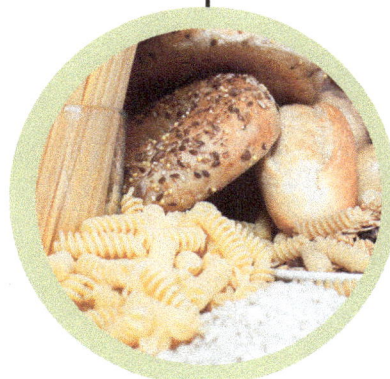

4 Carbohydrates

Cravings for carbs can be an indicator of low serotonin. Choose complex carbs and pair them with healthy fat and protein. Carbohydrate cravings may be related to lack of sleep.

What Else is it Saying...

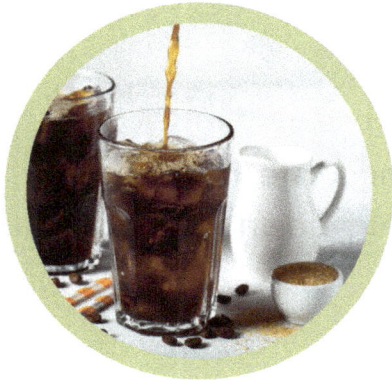

5 Caffeine

Craving caffeine is a sign that you need an energy boost. It could also indicate low iron.

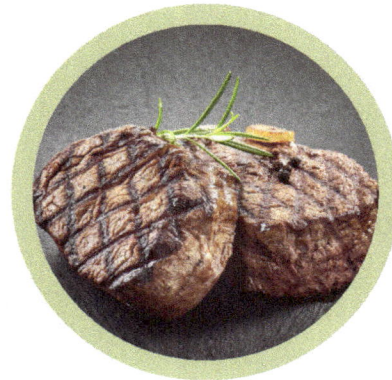

6 Red Meat

Craving red meat can be an indicator of a deficiency in iron, vitamin B, and zinc.

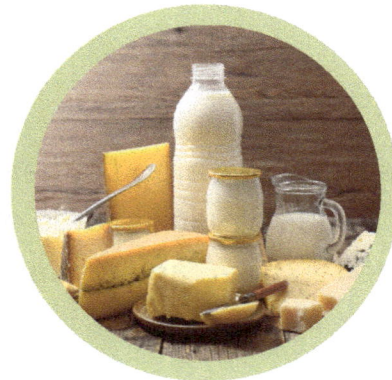

7 Dairy

A craving for dairy could suggest a need for calcium or healthy fats.

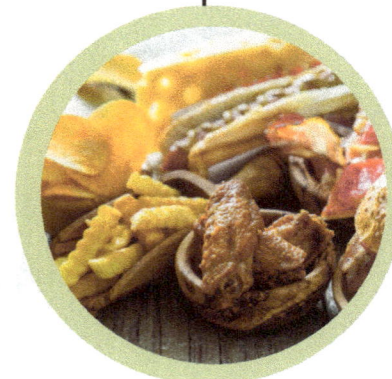

8 Fatty Foods

Craving fatty foods could be an indicator that you need healthy fats like Omega-3.

Switch it up

Now that you know what your body is trying to tell you, what can you switch up when craving unhealthy foods? Be sure to track how you feel after switching it up.

Instead of chocolate, I need to eat leafy greens, nuts, legumes,

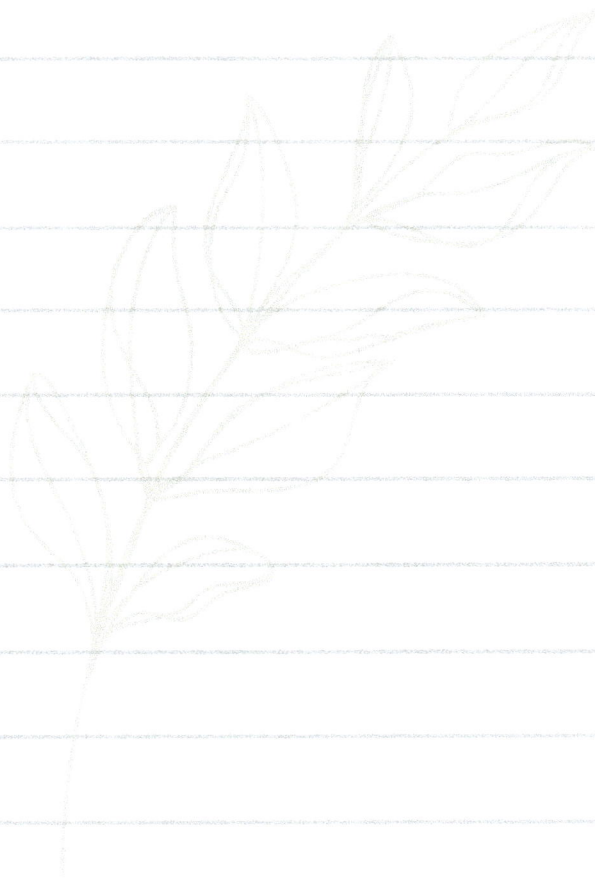

Eat Healthy

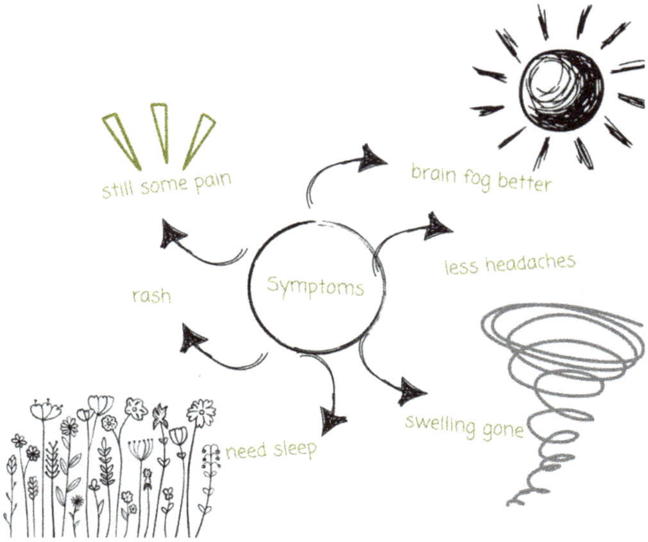

Track It!

Feel free to use the lines on this page to jot down your symptoms, mood, or anything else that comes to mind— or you could even doodle it!

still some pain

brain fog better

rash

Symptoms

less headaches

need sleep

swelling gone

Track It

Reflection Time

What is your soul craving?

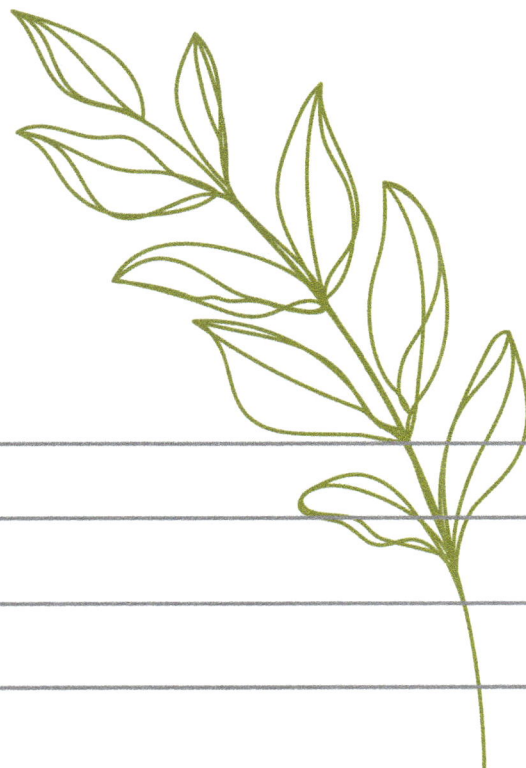

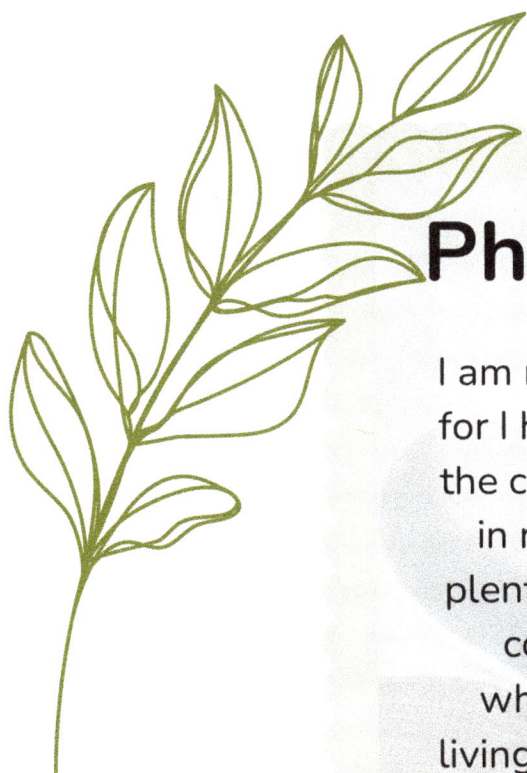

_____

_____

_____

_____

Philippians 4:11-13

I am not saying this because I am in need, for I have learned to be content whatever the circumstances. I know what it is to be in need, and I know what it is to have plenty. I have learned the secret of being content in any and every situation, whether well fed or hungry, whether living in plenty or in want. I can do all this through him who gives me strength.

God's Word

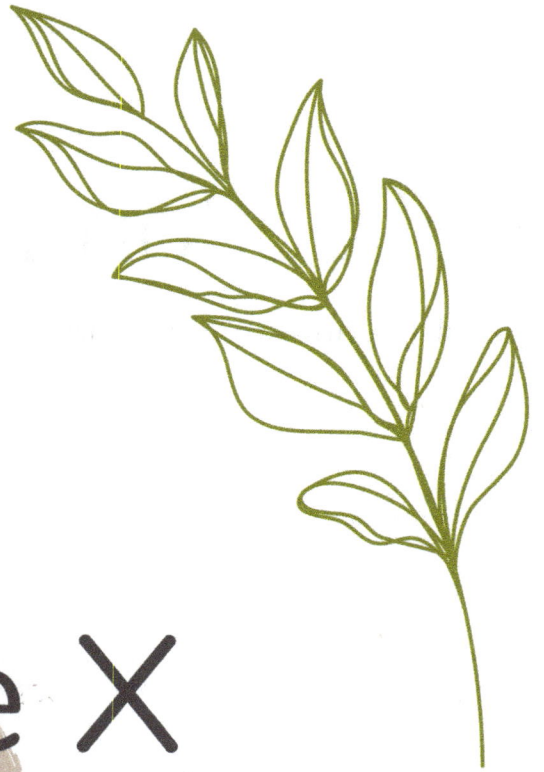

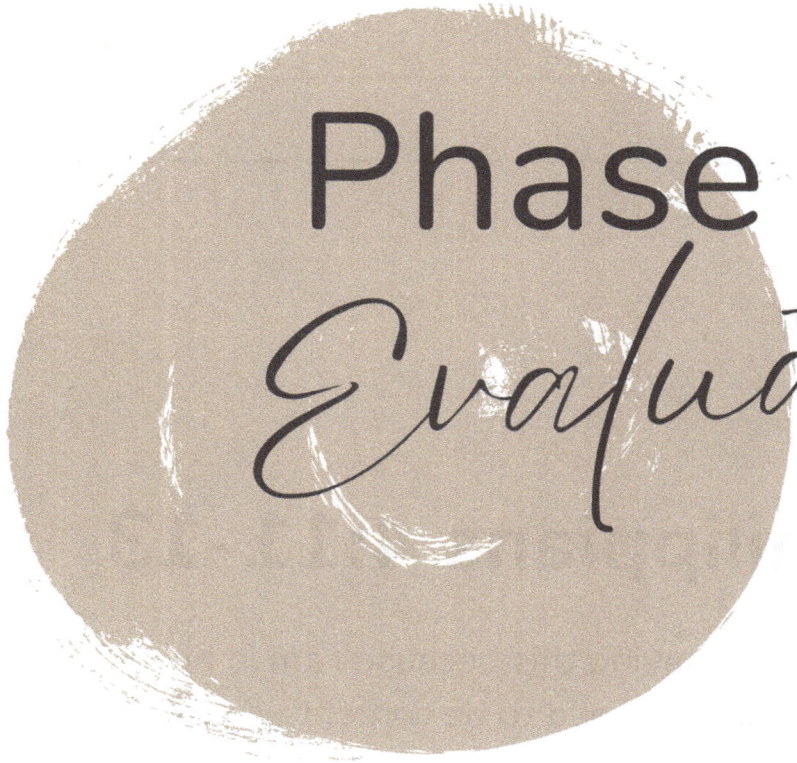

Phase X
Evaluate

Check In

It's time to evaluate how you are doing. Let's reflect on what progress you have made. Jot your progress for each topic.

Reduce Inflammation

New Ways

Sleep

Water Intake

Take it up a Notch

Balance Blood Sugar

How'd you do?

Follow up on the Process

What do you feel didn't work for you? Keeping track will help you to move forward.

What wins did you have during this?

DIDN'T WORK:

WORKED:

Symptom Check

Compare your current symptoms with the ones from the beginning of your healing journey.

Then

- ☐ Chronic Fatigue
- ☐ Unexplained Pain
- ☐ Digestive Issues
- ☐ Brain Fog
- ☐ Headaches and Migraines
- ☐ Skin Problems
- ☐ Sleep Disturbance

Now

- ☐ Chronic Fatigue
- ☐ Unexplained Pain
- ☐ Digestive Issues
- ☐ Brain Fog
- ☐ Headaches and Migraines
- ☐ Skin Problems
- ☐ Sleep Disturbance

Any other symptoms still lingering?

More Details...

We still have some changes to explore, so if you are still experiencing symptoms, do not get discouraged.

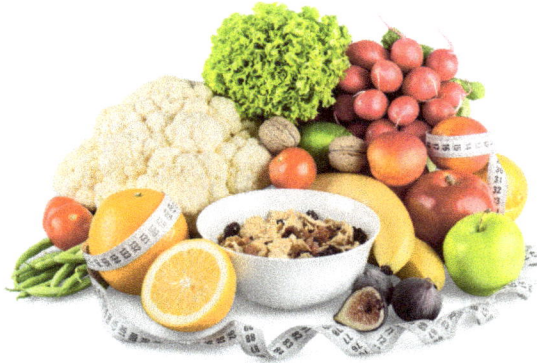

The following pages offer introductory steps to healing based on your symptoms. The table allows you to easily navigate the resource and select your specific symptoms.

SYMPTOM DIET

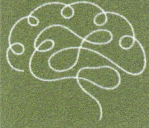

Brain Fog and Cognitive Issues

- Possible causes: Poor diet, nutrient deficiencies, inflammation, hormonal imbalances
- Dietary solutions:
  - Prioritize foods rich in antioxidants and brain-boosting nutrients such as omega-3 fatty acids (found in fatty fish, flaxseeds, and chia seeds), berries, leafy greens, and nuts.
  - Include sources of choline (found in eggs, liver, and cruciferous vegetables) and phospholipids (found in soy lecithin, eggs, and organ meats) to support cognitive function.
  - Avoid processed foods, refined sugars, and artificial additives that can contribute to brain fog and inflammation.

Digestive Issues (Bloating, Gas, Constipation, Diarrhea)

- Possible causes: Food sensitivities, inadequate fiber intake, imbalanced gut microbiota
- Dietary solutions:
  - Keep a food diary to identify trigger foods and consider elimination diets to pinpoint problem foods.
  - Increase fiber intake through fruits, vegetables, whole grains, and legumes to support digestive health.
  - Consider probiotic-rich foods like yogurt, kefir, sauerkraut, and kombucha to promote a healthy gut microbiome.
  - Consider Food Combining to assist with digestion.

Fatigue

- Possible causes:
  - Imbalanced blood sugar levels
  - Nutrient deficiencies
  - Poor diet choices
- Dietary solutions:
  - Opt for balanced meals containing complex carbohydrates, lean proteins, and healthy fats to stabilize blood sugar levels.
  - Include energy-boosting foods like whole grains, nuts, seeds, and leafy greens in your diet.
  - Avoid sugary snacks and processed foods that can lead to energy crashes.

SYMPTOM DIET CONT...

Food Sensitivities and Allergies

- Possible causes: Undetected sensitivities or allergies to certain foods
- Dietary solutions:
  - Work with a healthcare professional to identify trigger foods through elimination-challenge testing.
  - Avoid common allergens such as gluten, dairy, soy, and nuts if sensitivities are suspected.
  - Experiment with alternative ingredients and allergen-free recipes to enjoy a diverse and satisfying diet.

Inflammation and Pain

- Possible causes: Poor dietary choices, chronic stress, underlying health conditions
- Dietary solutions:
  - Focus on an anti-inflammatory diet rich in omega-3 fatty acids (found in fatty fish, flaxseeds, and walnuts), antioxidants (found in colorful fruits and vegetables), and spices like turmeric and ginger.
  - Limit intake of inflammatory foods such as refined sugars, processed meats, and trans fats.
  - Stay hydrated with plenty of water and herbal teas to flush out toxins and reduce inflammation.

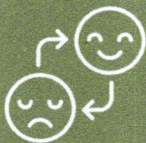

Mood Swings

- Possible causes: Imbalanced neurotransmitters, blood sugar fluctuations, nutrient deficiencies
- Dietary solutions:
  - Incorporate mood-boosting foods rich in tryptophan (found in turkey, chicken, bananas, and dairy), magnesium (found in leafy greens, nuts, seeds, and legumes), and complex carbohydrates (found in whole grains, fruits, and vegetables).
  - Focus on regular, balanced meals to stabilize blood sugar levels and support emotional well-being.
  - Limit caffeine and alcohol intake, as they can exacerbate mood swings and disrupt sleep patterns.

Nutrient Deficiencies

- Possible causes: Malabsorption issues, dietary restrictions, increased nutrient demands
- Dietary solutions:
  - Incorporate nutrient-dense foods such as fruits, vegetables, whole grains, lean proteins, and healthy fats into your diet.
  - Consider supplementation under the guidance of a healthcare professional to address specific nutrient deficiencies.
  - Aim for a well-rounded diet that provides essential vitamins and minerals to support overall health and well-being.

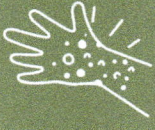

Skin Issues (psoriasis, eczema, acne)

- Possible causes: Inflammation, food sensitivities, imbalanced gut microbiota
- Dietary solutions:
  - Adopt an anti-inflammatory diet rich in fruits, vegetables, healthy fats, and lean proteins to support skin health.
  - Consider eliminating common trigger foods such as dairy, gluten, and processed sugars to see if symptoms improve.
  - Increase intake of foods high in vitamins A, C, and E (found in carrots, sweet potatoes, citrus fruits, nuts, and seeds) to promote skin healing and regeneration.

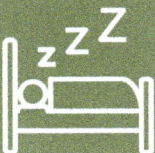

Sleep Disturbance and Insomnia

- Possible causes: Disrupted circadian rhythm, stress, imbalanced neurotransmitters
- Dietary solutions:
  - Establish a bedtime routine and avoid heavy meals, caffeine, and alcohol close to bedtime.
  - Include sleep-promoting foods rich in tryptophan (found in turkey, chicken, dairy, and bananas) and magnesium (found in nuts, seeds, leafy greens, and legumes) in your evening meals or snacks.
  - Experiment with herbal teas such as chamomile, valerian root, or passionflower to promote relaxation and improve sleep quality.

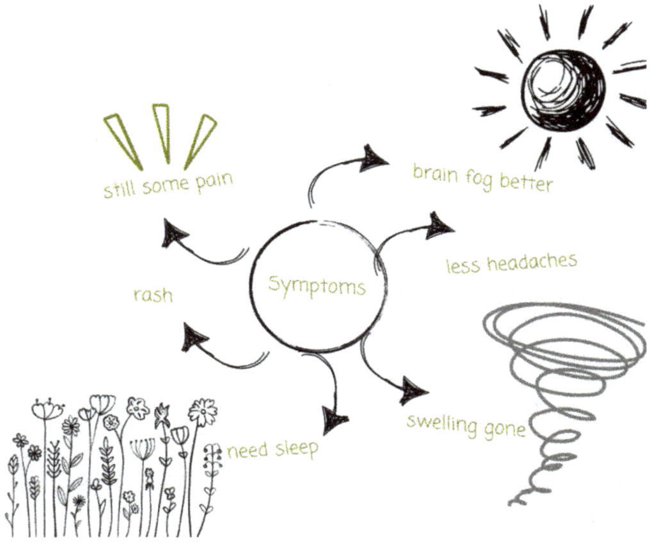

still some pain

brain fog better

rash

Symptoms

less headaches

need sleep

swelling gone

Track It!

Feel free to use the lines on this page to jot down your symptoms, mood, or anything else that comes to mind— or you could even doodle it!

Track It

Reflection Time

Examine my heart, Lord, and test my mind;
Reveal the paths I've walked, the truth I may find.
In the mirror of Your wisdom, my actions align,
Guide me to growth, in Your light I'll shine.

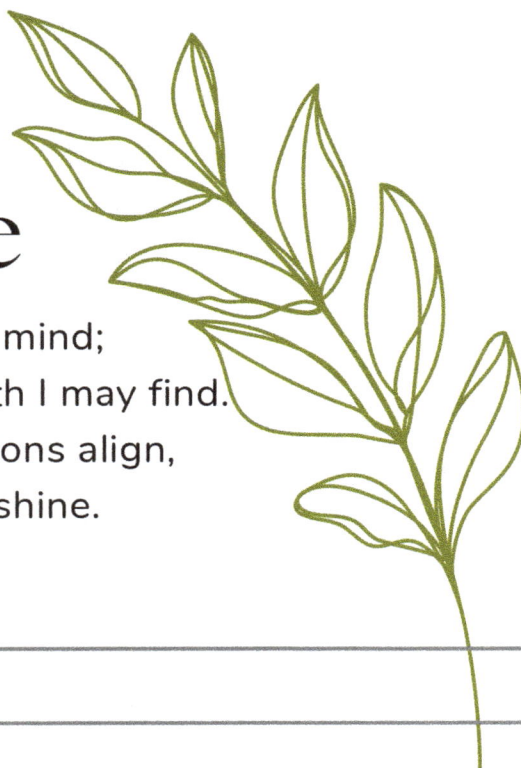

_____

_____

_____

_____

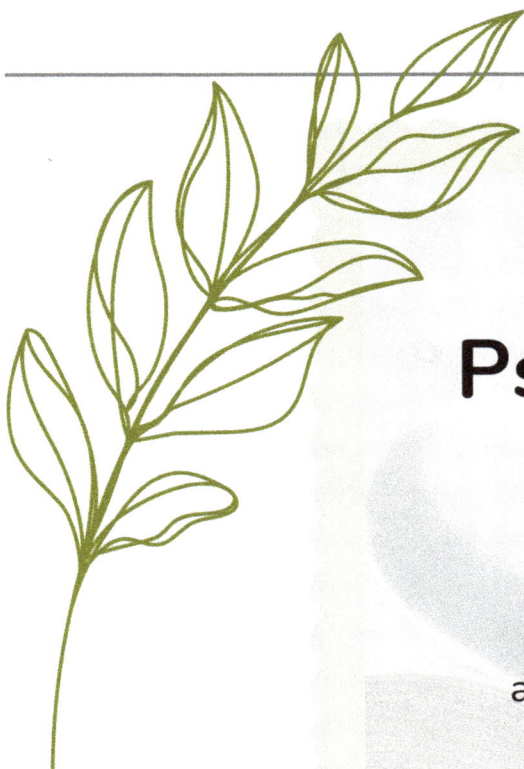

Psalm 139:23-24

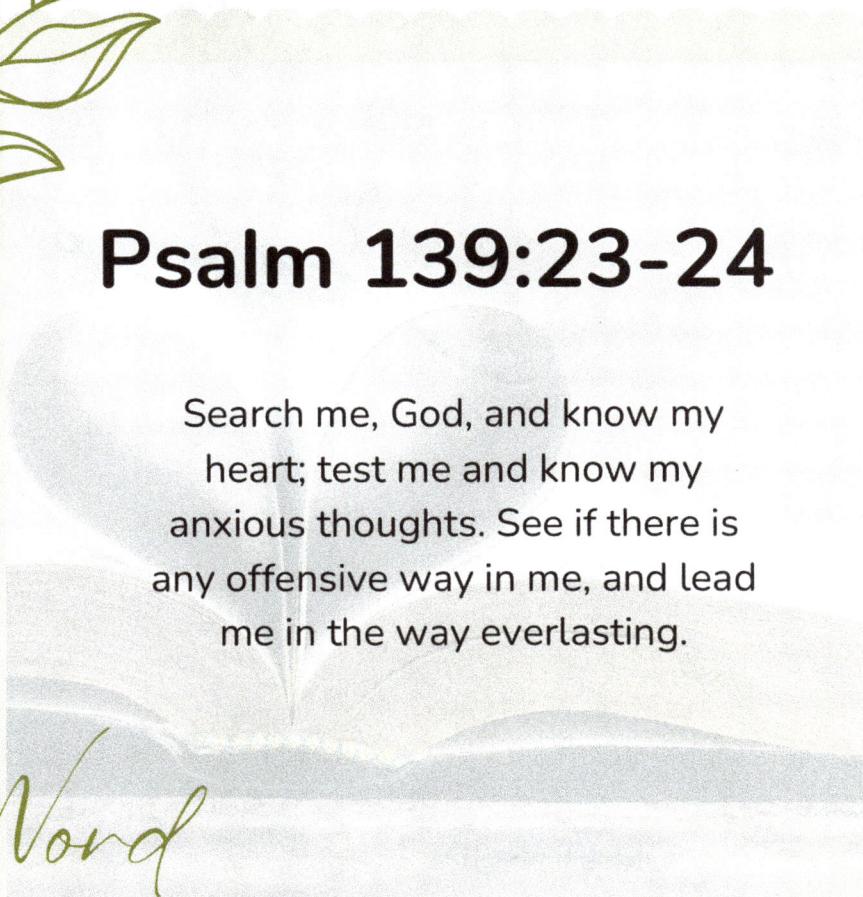

Search me, God, and know my
heart; test me and know my
anxious thoughts. See if there is
any offensive way in me, and lead
me in the way everlasting.

God's Word

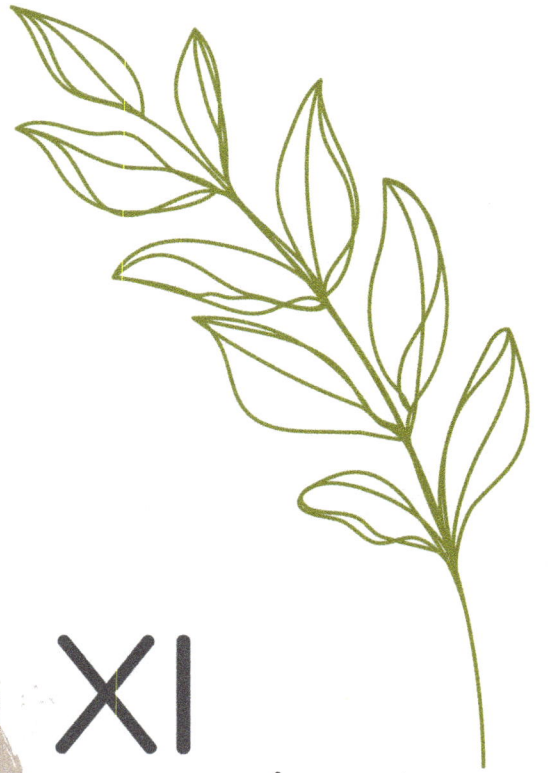

Phase XI
Nutrient Dense

Where are you on the nutrient dense path?

We've made a lot of changes on this journey, so let's keep taking those baby steps forward. Circle where you are and commit to moving to the next level.

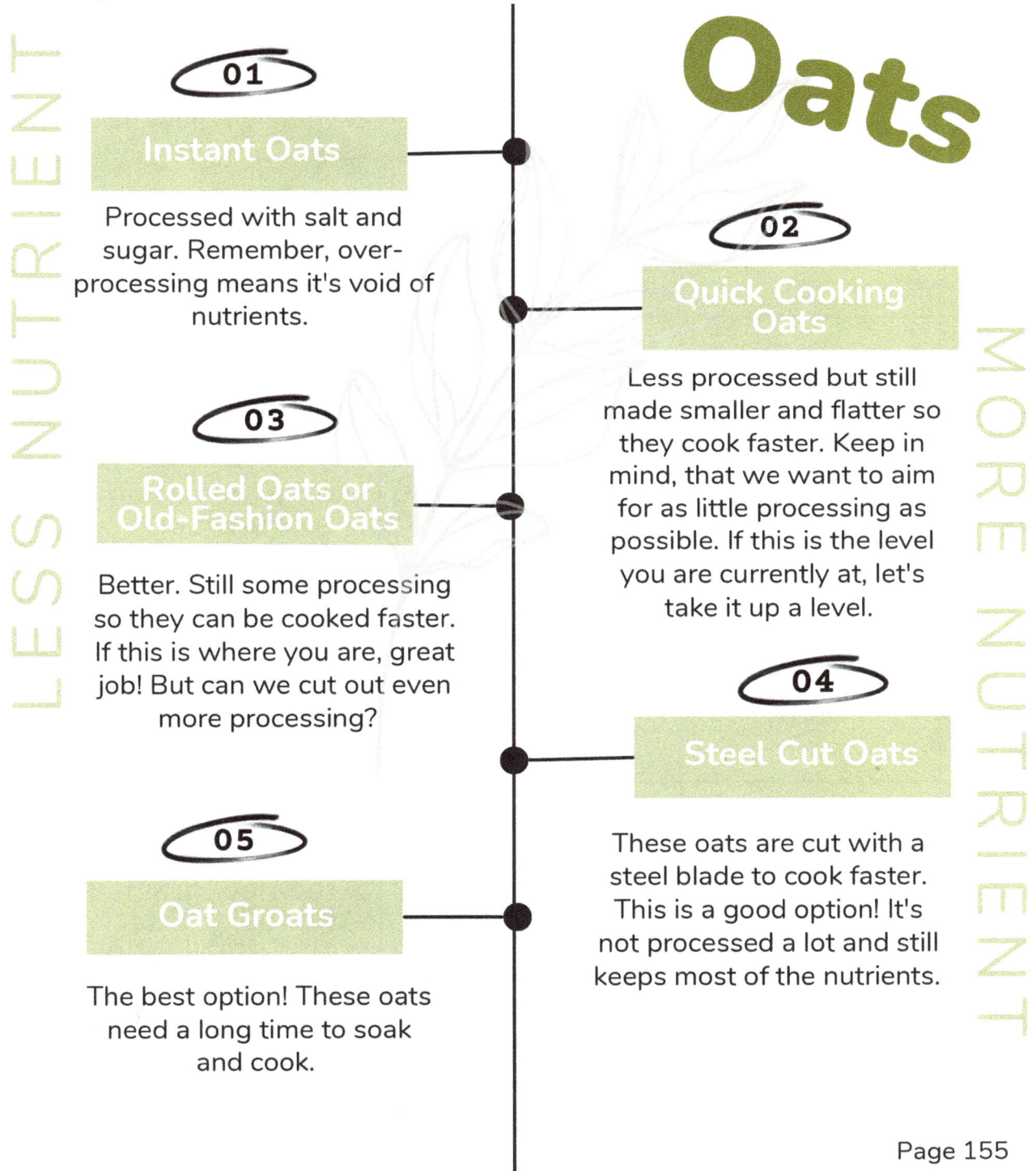

Oats

LESS NUTRIENT

MORE NUTRIENT

01 — Instant Oats

Processed with salt and sugar. Remember, over-processing means it's void of nutrients.

02 — Quick Cooking Oats

Less processed but still made smaller and flatter so they cook faster. Keep in mind, that we want to aim for as little processing as possible. If this is the level you are currently at, let's take it up a level.

03 — Rolled Oats or Old-Fashion Oats

Better. Still some processing so they can be cooked faster. If this is where you are, great job! But can we cut out even more processing?

04 — Steel Cut Oats

These oats are cut with a steel blade to cook faster. This is a good option! It's not processed a lot and still keeps most of the nutrients.

05 — Oat Groats

The best option! These oats need a long time to soak and cook.

Where are you on the nutrient dense path?

How about wheat? Each one of these changes increases nutrient intake. Mark which changes you will try first and make a commitment to better choices.

Wheat

Ok	Better	Tips
White Rice	Brown Rice	Start with brown basmati rice, then short grain brown rice.
Wheat	Whole Grain	Mix whole grain to transition. Only eat wheat if your body tolerates.
Pasta	Garbanzo, Quinoa, Brown Rice Pasta	Watch for corn additives.
Rice	Millet	Mix millet with rice to introduce the new grain gradually. Start with a small ratio.
Pancakes	Buckwheat Pancakes	Start with a 50/50 blend.

LESS NUTRIENT

MORE NUTRIENT

More Detail...

Why are these changes important? Let's first look at the process of wheat and then you can decide why. Then look at the impact you can make just by adding more nutrient-dense foods into your diet.

HOW WHEAT IS PROCESSED

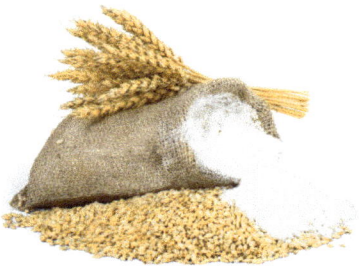

While you may not have a gluten sensitivity, it's essential to understand the broader implications of chemical processing in wheat. Let's uncover the hidden impacts of chemical exposure in wheat production.

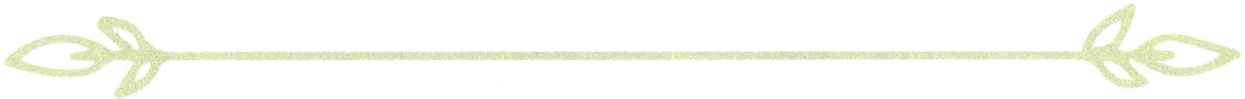

How Wheat is Processed

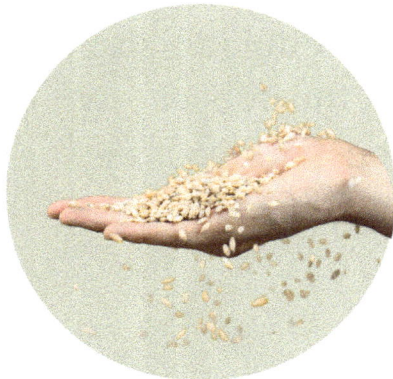

1 Seed Preparation

Before farmers plant wheat, they treat the seeds with chemicals to protect them from bugs and fungi. It's like giving the seeds a little shield.

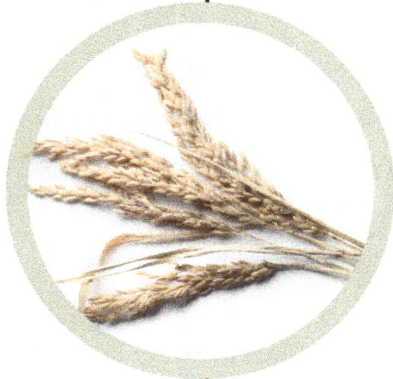

2 Stalk

As the wheat plant grows, they add synthetic growth regulators to guide how it grows. It's like giving the plant a little nudge to grow the way they want.

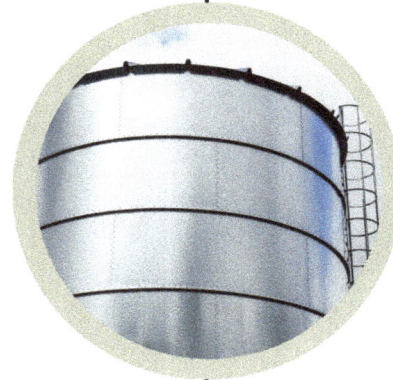

3 Grain Storage

In the grain storage phase, insecticides make a return, accompanied by possible fumigation to protect against pests.

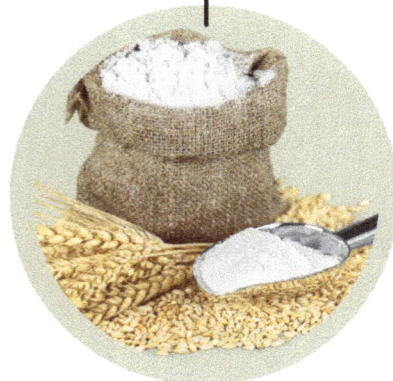

4 Milling and Processing

During milling, high-energy radiation becomes a tool to remove bran and germ, shaping the characteristics of the resulting flour.

There are three parts to the grain:

1. **Bran** - fiber-rich outer layer that supplies B vitamins, iron, copper, zinc, magnesium, antioxidants, and phytochemicals.

2. **Germ** - rich in healthy fats, vitamin E, B vitamins, phytochemicals and antioxidants

3. **Endosperm** - carbohydrates, protein, and small amounts of some B vitamins and minerals. Gluten is concentrated in the endosperm.

During the milling process of grains like wheat, the bran and germ are often removed, leaving behind the endosperm, which contains gluten. For individuals with gluten sensitivity or celiac disease, consuming gluten can trigger an immune response that damages the lining of the small intestine, leading to difficulty absorbing nutrients.

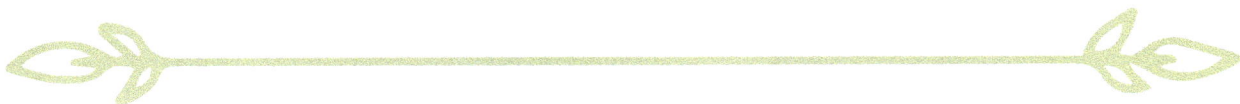

NUTRIENT DENSE

Discover the power of nutrient-dense foods—those rich in vitamins, minerals, fiber, and protein, offering maximum nutrition with fewer calories. We'll explore how foods like leafy greens, whole grains, and healthy fats support better digestion, stable energy, and disease prevention, while also helping with weight management.

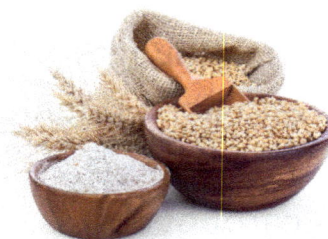

WHAT IS NUTRIENT-DENSE?

When we refer to nutrient-dense foods, we're talking about foods that provide a high amount of essential nutrients relative to their calorie content. These nutrients include vitamins, minerals, fiber, protein, healthy fats, and antioxidants. Essentially, nutrient-dense foods pack a lot of nutritional value into each calorie, helping you meet your daily nutritional needs without consuming excessive calories.

Characteristics of Nutrient-Dense Foods:

High in Vitamins and Minerals: These foods are rich in essential nutrients like vitamin C, vitamin A, B vitamins, calcium, iron, magnesium, and potassium, which your body needs to function optimally.

Rich in Fiber: Fiber helps with digestion, supports gut health, stabilizes blood sugar, and can aid in weight management. Nutrient-dense foods tend to be high in fiber.

Good Source of Healthy Fats and Protein: They provide good-quality proteins and healthy fats, which are important for muscle repair, brain function, and long-lasting energy.

Low in Empty Calories: Nutrient-dense foods have fewer empty calories (calories that provide no nutritional benefit), such as added sugars and unhealthy fats.

Lower in Refined or Processed Ingredients: They are often whole foods or minimally processed, which means they retain more of their natural nutrients compared to highly processed foods.

Examples

Healthy fats like avocados, nuts, seeds, olive oil, and fatty fish (like salmon) provide heart-healthy fats, omega-3 fatty acids, and fat-soluble vitamins making them nutrient-dense. Here are some more examples of nutrient-dense foods:

Leafy Greens

Spinach, kale, Swiss chard, and arugula are loaded with vitamins (especially A, C, and K), minerals, and fiber.

Fruits

Berries (blueberries, raspberries, strawberries), citrus fruits, and apples are rich in vitamins, antioxidants, and fiber.

Vegetables

Broccoli, Brussels sprouts, sweet potatoes, carrots, and bell peppers are packed with essential nutrients.

Whole Grains

Brown rice, quinoa, oats, and millet provide fiber, protein, and a range of vitamins and minerals.

Lean Protein

Chicken, turkey, beans, lentils, and tofu are excellent sources of protein and other nutrients like iron and B vitamins.

Legumes

Beans, lentils, and chickpeas offer a mix of protein, fiber, and complex carbohydrates.

Nutrient Dense

Benefits

More Nutrients = Greater Satiety (Fullness)

Increased Nutrient Density = Fewer Calories

Improved Digestive Health

More Stable Energy Levels

Better Long-Term Health

Nutrient-Rich Foods Support Immune Function

Improved Skin, Hair, and Nail Health

Reduced Inflammation

Healthy

Track It!

Feel free to use the lines on this page to jot down your symptoms, mood, or anything else that comes to mind— or you could even doodle it!

still some pain

brain fog better

rash

Symptoms

less headaches

need sleep

swelling gone

Track It

Reflection Time

Keep going! You got this!

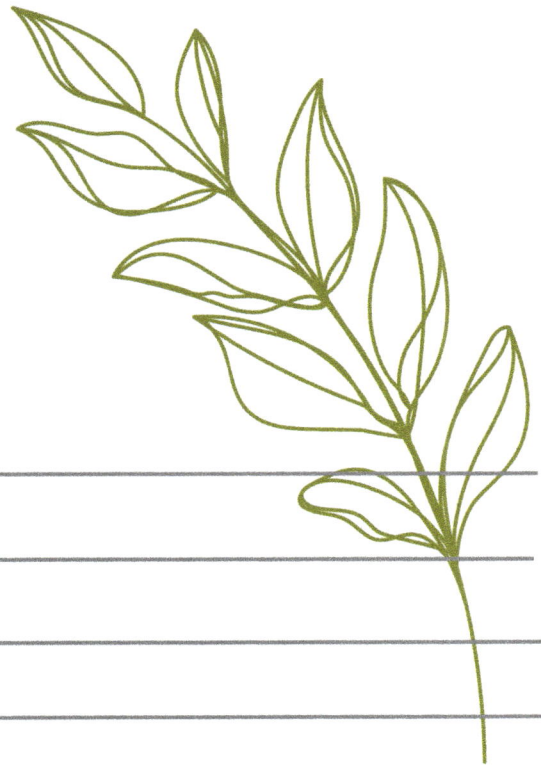

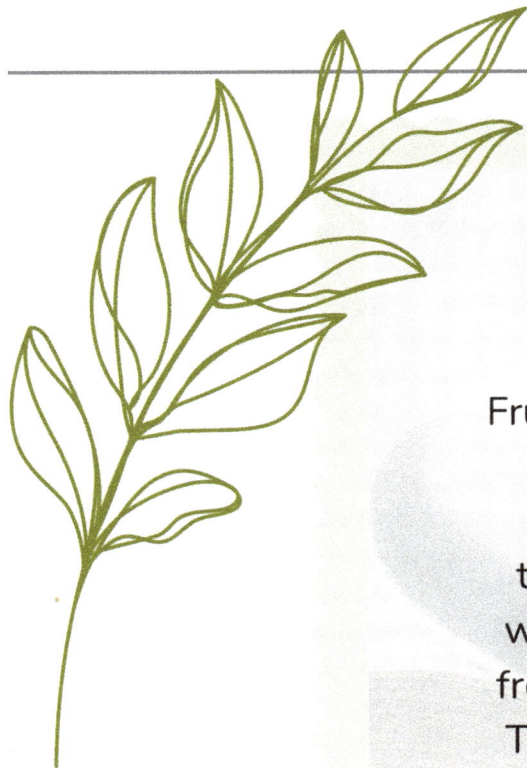

_____

_____

_____

_____

_____

_____

Ezekiel 47:12

Fruit trees of all kinds will grow on both banks of the river. Their leaves will not wither, nor will their fruit fail. Every month they will bear fruit, because the water from the sanctuary flows to them. Their fruit will serve for food and their leaves for healing.

God's Word

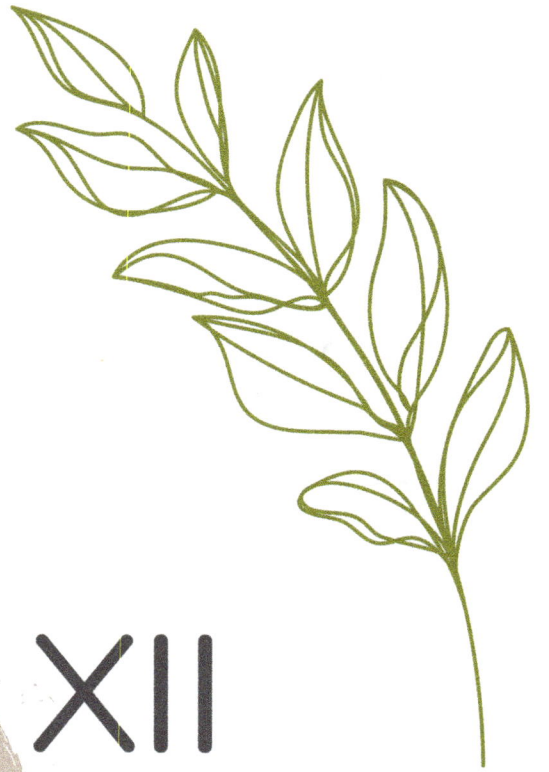

Phase XII

Toxins

What Toxins are in Your Home?

Toxins in the home wreak havoc on our bodies. Let's take inventory of your home to see what toxins you currently have in the home. Jot them down here.

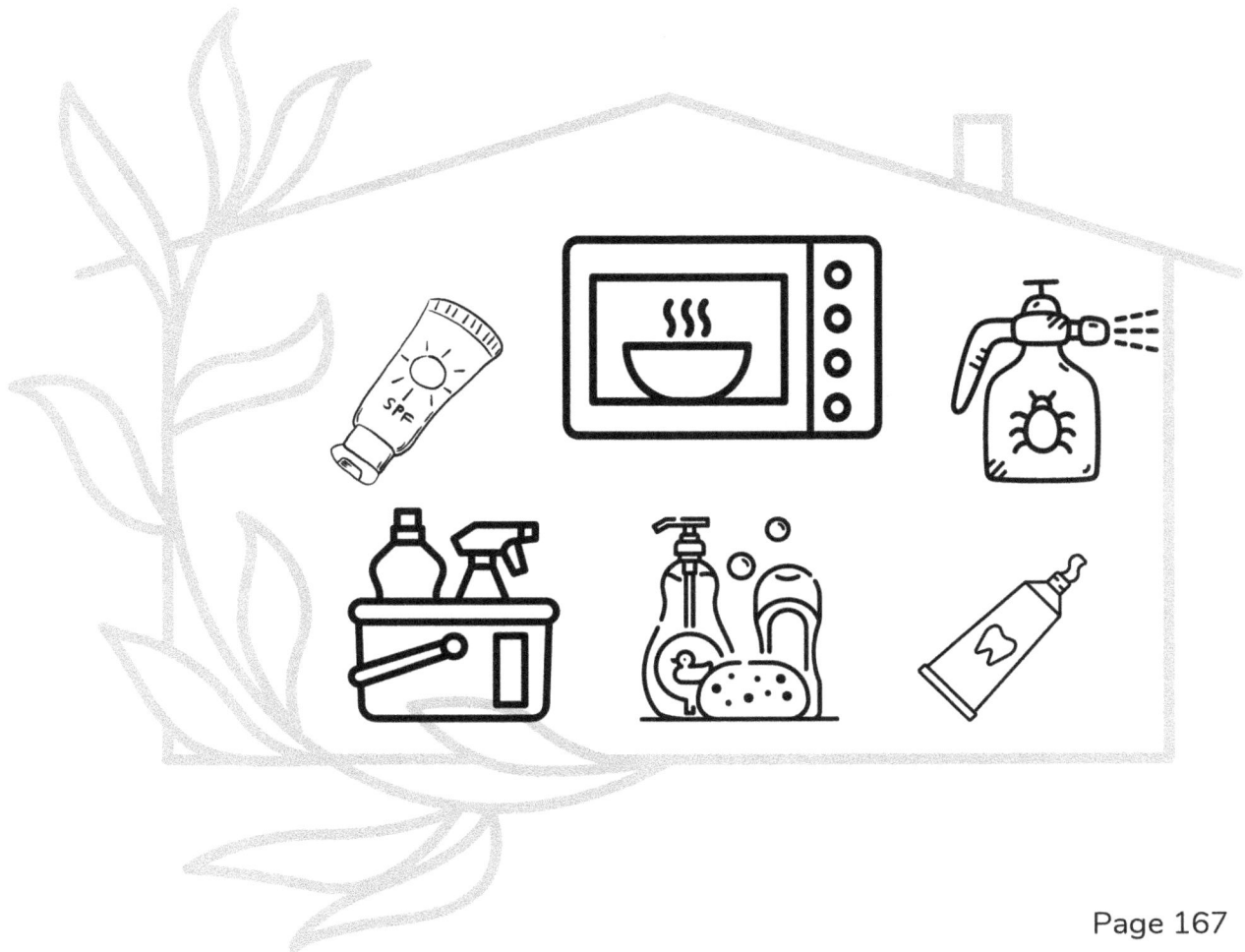

_____

_____

_____

_____

C H E C K L I S T

Did you consider these items too? Check off the items as you replace them with better options. It is impossible to remove all toxins from our environment, but we can at least try to remove as many as possible from our homes.

- [ ] ALL PURPOSE CLEANERS
- [ ] GLASS CLEANERS
- [ ] BATHROOM CLEANERS
- [ ] DISINFECTANTS
- [ ] FLOOR CLEANERS
- [ ] OVEN CLEANERS
- [ ] AIR FRESHENERS
- [ ] CANDLES
- [ ] LAUNDRY DETERGENT
- [ ] DISH SOAP

- [ ] CARPET CLEANER
- [ ] SHAMPOO
- [ ] CONDITIONER
- [ ] BODY WASHES AND SOAPS
- [ ] LOTIONS
- [ ] DEODORANT
- [ ] TOOHPASTE
- [ ] NAIL POLISH
- [ ] HAIR DYES
- [ ] SUNSCREEN

To Remove

More Details...

REPLACING TOXINS

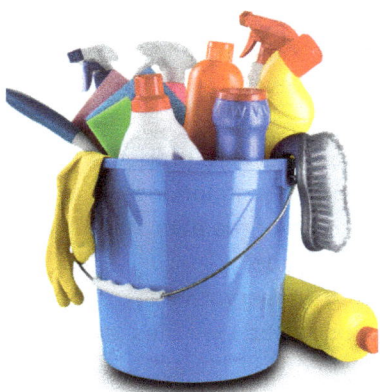

Explore the hidden toxins lurking in everyday household products and how they impact your health. From cleaning supplies to personal care items, you'll learn to identify harmful ingredients and understand their potential long-term effects on your body. Discover practical, non-toxic alternatives that promote a cleaner, safer environment for you and your family.

Many common toxins found in cleaning and body care products can have harmful effects on the body over time. These chemicals can disrupt hormone function, and lead to issues like hormonal imbalances and fertility problems. Some toxins may irritate the skin, eyes, or respiratory system, causing allergic reactions, asthma, or dermatitis. Others are linked to long-term health concerns, such as cancer, neurological issues, and damage to organs like the liver or kidneys.

Additionally, exposure to certain toxins may contribute to the buildup of harmful substances in the body, impacting overall health and weakening the immune system.

By reducing exposure to these toxins, you can help protect your health and support your body's natural detoxification processes.

COMMON TOXIC INGREDIENTS

Household Cleaning Products	Body Care Products
1. Phthalates ○ **Found in:** Air fresheners, scented cleaners ○ **Watch for:** Fragrance, as phthalates are often hidden under this term **2. Triclosan** ○ **Found in:** Antibacterial cleaners ○ **Watch for:** Triclosan or "antibacterial" labels **3. Ammonia** ○ **Found in:** Window cleaners, oven cleaners, and polishes ○ **Watch for:** Ammonia on the label **4. Chlorine** ○ **Found in:** Bleach, toilet bowl cleaners, mildew removers ○ **Watch for:** Sodium hypochlorite or "bleach" on labels **5. Sodium Lauryl Sulfate (SLS)** ○ **Found in:** Detergents, all-purpose cleaners ○ **Watch for:** Sodium lauryl sulfate or sodium laureth sulfate **6. 2-Butoxyethanol** ○ **Found in:** Window cleaners, kitchen cleaners ○ **Watch for:** 2-butoxyethanol or ethylene glycol butyl ether **7. Quaternary Ammonium Compounds (Quats)** ○ **Found in:** Disinfecting sprays, fabric softeners ○ **Watch for:** Benzalkonium chloride or quaternary ammonium compounds	**1. Parabens** ○ **Found in:** Shampoos, lotions, and cosmetics ○ **Watch for:** Methylparaben, ethylparaben, propylparaben, butylparaben **2. Phthalates** ○ **Found in:** Scented personal care products like perfumes, deodorants, and lotions ○ **Watch for:** Fragrance, as phthalates are often hidden under this label **3. Formaldehyde-Releasing Preservatives** ○ **Found in:** Hair products, body washes, and lotions ○ **Watch for:** DMDM hydantoin, diazolidinyl urea, or imidazolidinyl urea **4. Triclosan** ○ **Found in:** Antibacterial soaps and toothpaste ○ **Watch for:** Triclosan on the ingredient list **5. Sodium Lauryl Sulfate (SLS)** ○ **Found in:** Shampoos, soaps, and toothpaste ○ **Watch for:** Sodium lauryl sulfate or sodium laureth sulfate **6. Toluene** ○ **Found in:** Nail polish, hair dye ○ **Watch for:** Toluene or benzene on the label **7. Oxybenzone** ○ **Found in:** Sunscreens ○ **Watch for:** Oxybenzone, benzophenone, or related compounds **8. Synthetic Fragrances** ○ **Found in:** Lotions, shampoos, deodorants, and perfumes ○ **Watch for:** "Fragrance" or "perfume," which can be a blend of harmful chemicals **9. Polyethylene Glycol (PEG)** ○ **Found in:** Creams, lotions, and cosmetics ○ **Watch for:** Ingredients labeled with PEG, such as PEG-8 or PEG-40 **10. DEA/TEA/MEA** ○ **Found in:** Soaps, shampoos, and lotions ○ **Watch for:** Diethanolamine (DEA), triethanolamine (TEA), or monoethanolamine (MEA)

REPLACEMENT CHALLENGE

Start to slowly replace your household cleaning products with non-toxic cleaning products. Eventually, you will feel and smell the difference in your home!

☑ **Remove:**   **Replacement:**

❖

☐ **Disinfectants**
1. Vinegar
   - Use as a natural disinfectant and cleaner for surfaces, glass, and mirrors
2. Hydrogen Peroxide
   - Use as a disinfectant for surfaces or to whiten laundry naturally

❖

☐ **Cleaner**
1. Baking Soda
   - Great for scrubbing sinks, tubs, and stovetops; neutralizes odors
2. Castile Soap
   - A gentle, plant-based soap that works well for cleaning floors, countertops, and even laundry
3. Microfiber Cloths
   - Use for dusting and cleaning without needing any chemical products

❖

☐ **Anti-bacterial**
1. Lemon Juice
   - Acts as a natural antibacterial agent and can help cut through grease

❖

☐ **Fresh scent**
1. Essential Oils (e.g., Tea Tree, Lavender, Lemon)
   - Can be added to homemade cleaners for a fresh scent and natural antibacterial properties

❖

☐ **Polish**
1. Olive Oil or Coconut Oil
   - Use as a furniture polish when mixed with a little lemon juice

❖

REPLACEMENT CHALLENGE

☑ Remove: **Replacement:**

---✤---

☐ Moisturizer

1. Coconut Oil
   - Can be used as a moisturizer, makeup remover, or hair conditioner.
2. Shea Butter
   - A natural, nourishing moisturizer for the skin.
3. Aloe Vera Gel
   - Soothes irritated skin, can be used as a light moisturizer or after-sun treatment.
4. Jojoba Oil or Argan Oil
   - Ideal for moisturizing skin and hair without clogging pores.
5. Avocado Oil
   - Natural

---✤---

☐ Toner

1. Apple Cider Vinegar
   - Works as a natural toner for the skin or a hair rinse to balance pH.
2. Witch Hazel
   - A natural astringent that can be used as a facial toner or to soothe irritated skin.

---✤---

☐ Bodywash and Shampoo

1. Castile Soap
   - A versatile, non-toxic body wash or shampoo alternative.

---✤---

☐ Deodorant

1. Baking Soda
   - Works as a natural deodorant when mixed with essential oils, or as a gentle exfoliant for the skin.
2. Homemade Deodorant
   - Made with ingredients like coconut oil, baking soda, and essential oils.

---✤---

☐ Toothpaste

1. Natural Toothpaste (Fluoride-Free)
   - Opt for fluoride-free or charcoal-based toothpaste without harmful additives.

---✤---

☐ Sunscreen

1. Mineral-based
   - Consider replacing with mineral-based sunscreens that use zinc oxide or titanium dioxide, which provide broad-spectrum protection without harmful chemicals.

2. Avocado Oil
   - Works as a natural SPF of approximately 4 to 15.

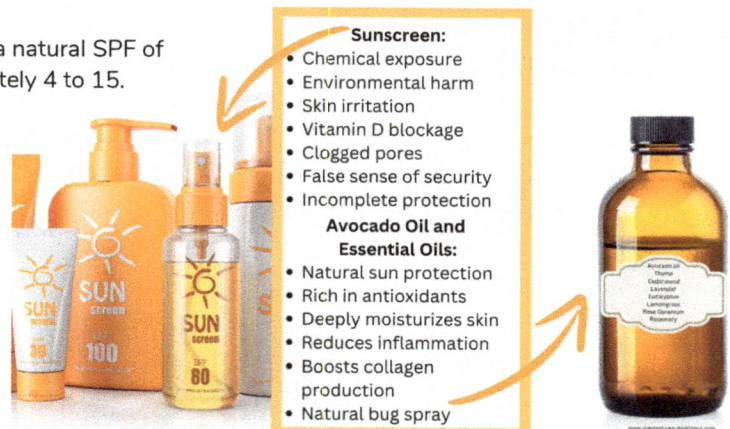

Sunscreen:
- Chemical exposure
- Environmental harm
- Skin irritation
- Vitamin D blockage
- Clogged pores
- False sense of security
- Incomplete protection

Avocado Oil and Essential Oils:
- Natural sun protection
- Rich in antioxidants
- Deeply moisturizes skin
- Reduces inflammation
- Boosts collagen production
- Natural bug spray

LOVE YOUR LIVER

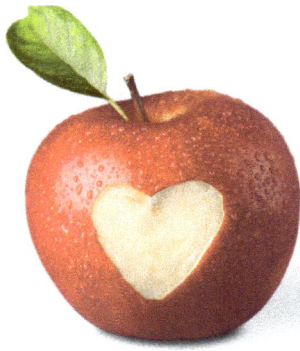

Your liver plays a vital role in maintaining your overall well-being. By understanding its functions, supporting it with a healthy lifestyle, and making mindful choices, you empower yourself to nurture a resilient and vibrant body.

9 things that can do harm to the liver over time:

Too much protein

Too much sugar and carbohydrates

Overeating

Drug residues

Too much enzyme deficient food

Inflammation from alcohol

Lack of exercise

Too many toxins, heavy metals, pesticides

Disease of liver (Hepatitis C)

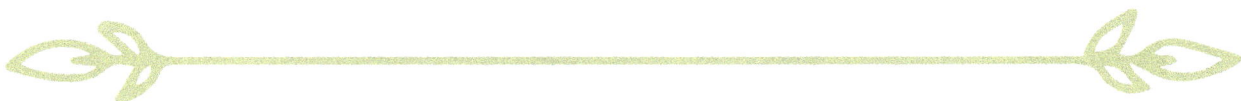

> "
> Stop harming your liver.
>
> Start helping your liver.
> "

Three ways to avoid toxins and help your liver:

Avoid microwaves

Choose organic

Refrain from plastic food containers

Avoid Toxins

> Leading sources of chlorinated pesticides are non-organic beef, non-organic dairy, farm-raised fish and non-organic butter.

Consider incorporating a liver-supporting supplement into your routine, but remember, it's essential to choose one that aligns with your preferences and needs. Conduct thorough research to find the supplement that resonates best with you and your health goals.

Detoxing Liver	Rebuild and Regenerate Liver
• Dandelion • Ginger • Cloves • Burdock Root • Horsetail	• Milk Thistle • Garlic • Dandelion • Wormwood • Black Walnut

Track It!

Feel free to use the lines on this page to jot down your symptoms, mood, or anything else that comes to mind— or you could even doodle it!

still some pain

brain fog better

rash

Symptoms

less headaches

need sleep

swelling gone

Track It

Reflection Time

Let's do our best to keep contaminates from our body and spirit.

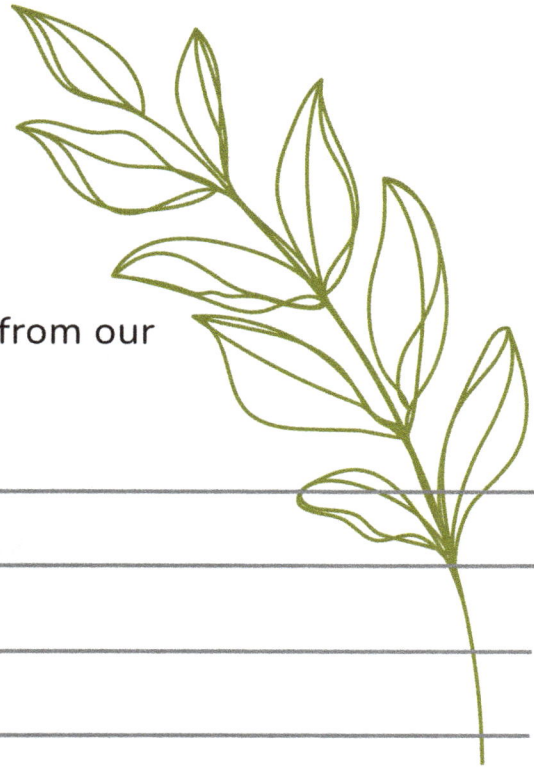

_____

_____

_____

_____

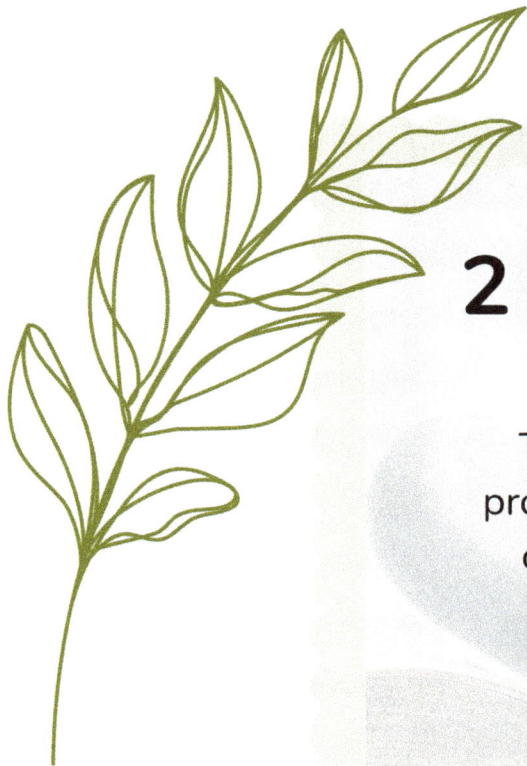

2 Corinthians 7:1

Therefore, since we have these promises, dear friends, let us purify ourselves from everything that contaminates body and spirit, perfecting holiness out of reverence for God.

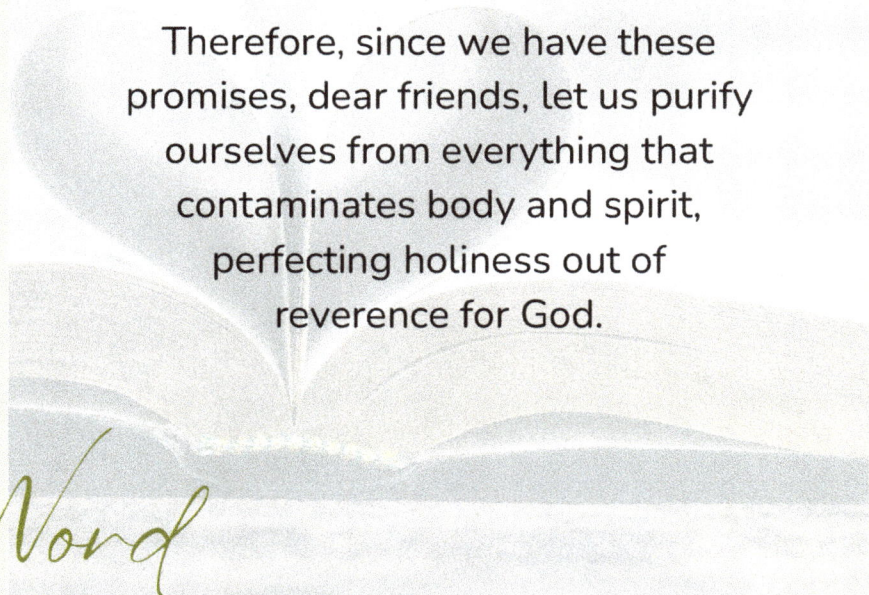

God's Word

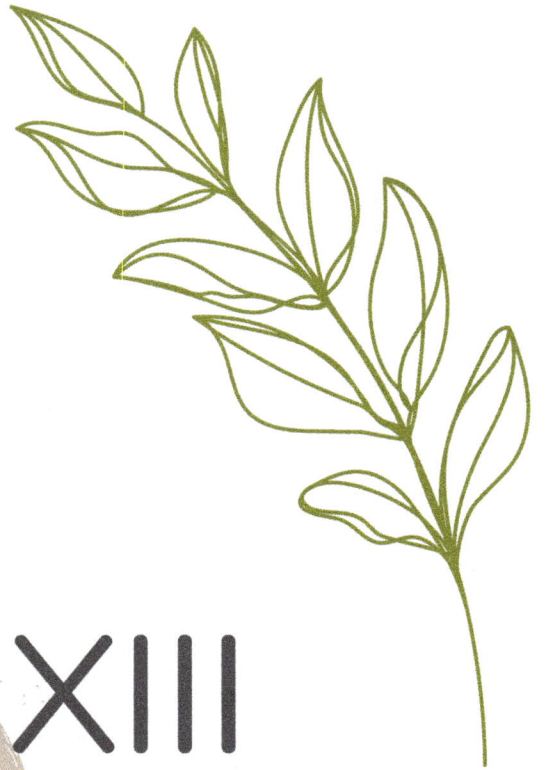

Phase XIII
Budget

Is it too expensive to eat healthy foods?

You may be asking how you can afford to eat healthier. Let's do a little activity to see where you currently stand with your budget.

Action Steps

1

Use the expense tracker to estimate your spending when you were eating out, fast foods, or cooking processed foods.

2

Use the 2nd expense tracker to estimate your spending now on whole foods.

3

Now add in your previous medical bills, missed work time, and put a price on your health.

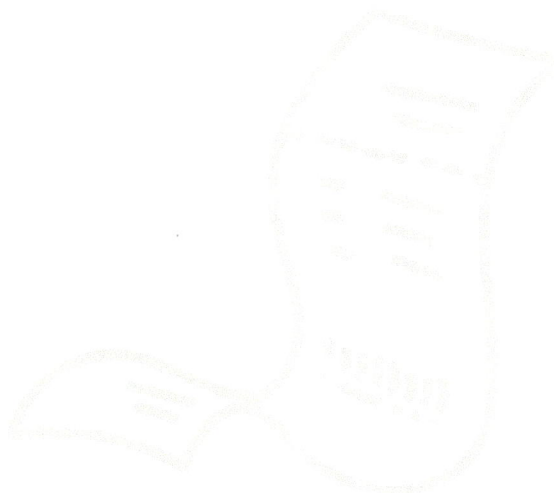

EXPENSE TRACKER

PROCESSED AND FAST FOODS

DATE	DESCRIPTION	CATEGORY	AMOUNT
			TOTAL

EXPENSE TRACKER

WHOLE FOODS

DATE	DESCRIPTION	CATEGORY	AMOUNT
		TOTAL	

TIPS

BUY FROZEN

Frozen fruits and vegetables can be more affordable and just as nutritious as fresh ones.

BUY IN BULK

Purchase non-perishable items like beans, rice, and oats in bulk. They have a longer shelf life and are often cheaper.

PLAN YOUR MEALS

Create a weekly meal plan to avoid impulse buys and food waste. Stick to your list when shopping.

COOK AT HOME

Preparing meals at home is generally more cost-effective than buying pre-packaged or restaurant food.

GROW YOUR OWN

Even a small container garden can save you money on herbs and some vegetables.

WHOLE CHICKEN

Whole chickens are often cheaper per pound than buying individual cuts. You can cook the whole chicken and use leftovers in various meals.

FREEZE OR CAN YOUR OWN

Freezing or canning your food is a cost-effective way to preserve seasonal produce and reduce waste. It allows you to enjoy fresh, healthy meals year-round while saving money and maintaining better control over ingredients and quality.

SHOP SEASONALLY

Buy fruits and vegetables that are in season as they tend to be cheaper and fresher.

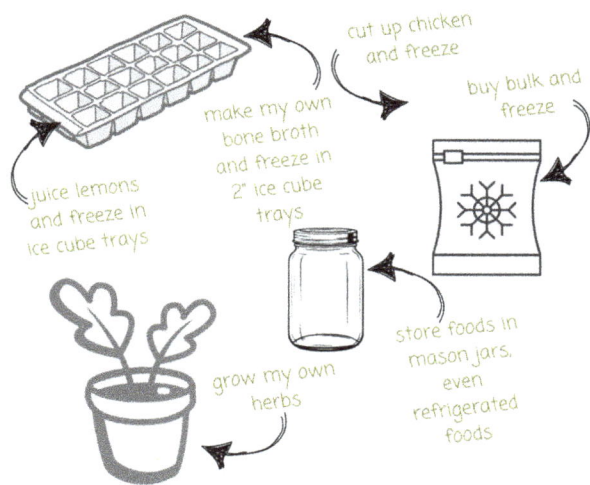

juice lemons
and freeze in
ice cube trays

make my own
bone broth
and freeze in
2" ice cube
trays

cut up chicken
and freeze

buy bulk and
freeze

store foods in
mason jars,
even
refrigerated
foods

grow my own
herbs

Brain Storm

Feel free to use the lines on this page to jot down your ideas to cut costs— or you could even doodle it!

Brain Storm

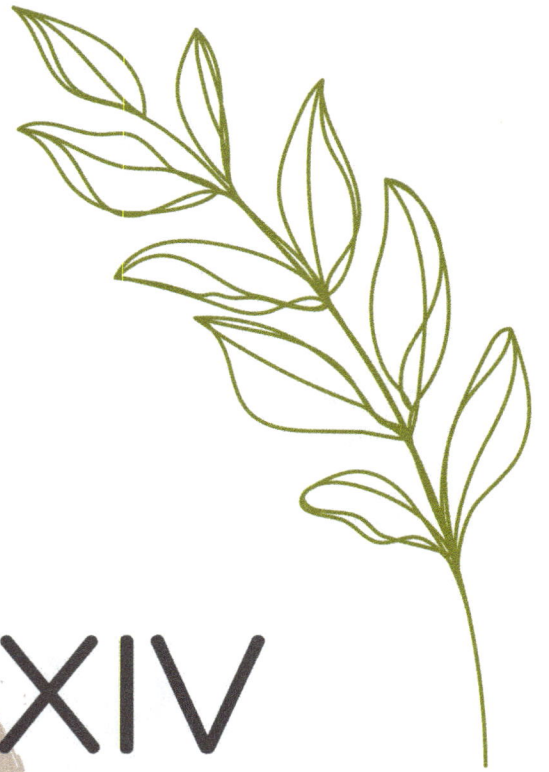

Phase XIV
Wrap it up

Thank you!

I appreciate your purchase of this book and commitment to better health. I am proud of you for taking the important steps towards healing. My hope and prayer for you is that you continue on this path and find ways to make it your lifestyle. Remember, you are not alone in this journey. Email me at any time. I would be happy to answer any questions or provide any additional tips.

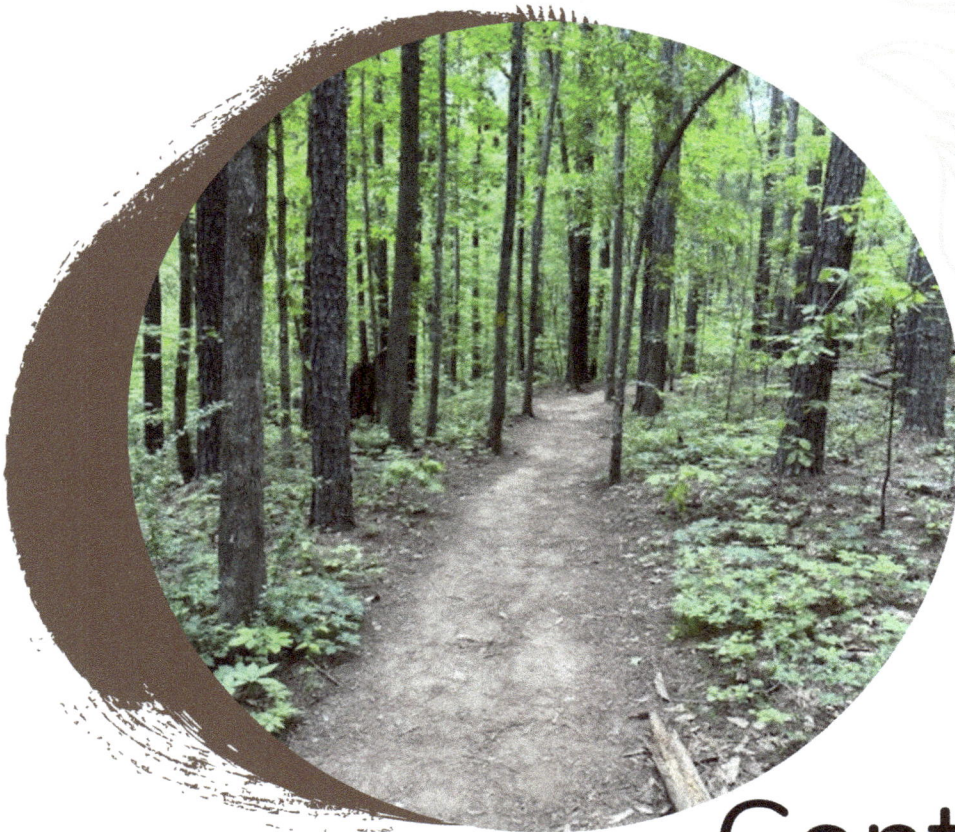

Contact:

Jsmith@supportivegutwellness.com

AUTHOR'S NOTE

My goal in writing this book is to make functional nutrition principles more accessible to everyone, whether you're dealing with chronic illness or simply looking to optimize your health. Through my personal experience and the work I completed while obtaining my certification in functional nutrition, I've seen how personalized nutrition can transform lives, and I'm eager to share that knowledge with you.

Please note that while the information in this book is based on evidence-based practices, it is not intended to replace personalized medical advice. I encourage you to consult with your healthcare provider before making any significant changes to your diet or lifestyle.

Finally, I'd like to express my gratitude to my many friends and family members, especially my daughters and grandsons. Their influence is woven into the pages of this book, and I am deeply thankful for the feedback and encouragement they've given me.

Jacqueline Smith

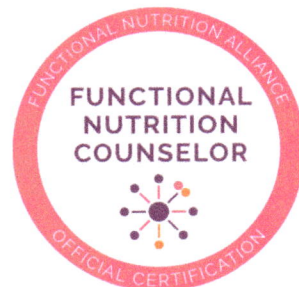

FUNCTIONAL
NUTRITION
COUNSELOR

FUNCTIONAL NUTRITION ALLIANCE

OFFICIAL CERTIFICATION

www.supportivegutwellness.com

ACKNOWLEDEMENT AND REFERENCES

Many of the concepts and resources in this book have been adapted from the teachings of Andrea Nakayama through the Functional Nutrition Alliance. I am deeply grateful for the education and insights provided during my training, which have shaped much of the information presented here.

For further learning and exploration, please visit the Functional Nutrition Alliance website at functionalnutritionlab.com.

Functional Nutrition. (n.d.). Image of gluten chart [Image]. Functional Nutrition. Retrieved from https://www.functionalnutrition.com

Fullscript. (n.d.). Image of processed food [Image]. Fullscript. Retrieved from https://www.fullscript.com

Fullscript. (n.d.). Image of circadian rhythm [Image]. Fullscript. Retrieved from https://www.fullscript.com

Fullscript. (n.d.). Image of creating an optimal sleep environment [Image]. Fullscript. Retrieved from https://www.fullscript.com

Fullscript. (n.d.). Image of essential oils for sleep [Image]. Fullscript. Retrieved from https://www.fullscript.com

DISCLAIMER

The information provided in this book is for educational and informational purposes only. It is based on the author's certification as a Functional Nutrition Coach, research, education, personal experience, and the integration of artificial intelligence (AI) tools. This book is not intended as a substitute for professional medical advice, diagnosis, or treatment.

The content reflects the principles of functional nutrition, but individual needs may vary. Readers should consult with a qualified healthcare provider, such as a licensed physician, registered dietitian, or nutritionist, before making any significant changes to their diet, lifestyle, or treatment plans. The author and publisher expressly disclaim responsibility for any adverse effects or consequences resulting from the use of the information in this book.

As a certified Functional Nutrition Coach, the author provides guidance on nutrition and wellness but does not diagnose, treat, cure, or prevent any medical conditions. Any products, services, or AI tools referenced in this book are for informational purposes only and do not constitute endorsements or guarantees.

While every effort has been made to ensure the accuracy of the information at the time of publication, the author and publisher make no representations or warranties regarding the completeness or current relevance of the content.

Please visit www.supportivegutwellness.com/supplements for important information on who should avoid certain supplements.